*Hospice and
Palliative Nurses Association*

MONOGRAPH

TREATMENT OF END-STAGE NON-CANCER DIAGNOSES

Hospice and Palliative Nurses Association Monograph
Treatment of End-Stage Non-Cancer Diagnoses

Volume IV Summer 2001

Published by
Hospice and Palliative Nurses Association
Penn Center West One, Suite 229
Pittsburgh, PA 15276

Copyright © 2001 by the Hospice and Palliative Nurses Association.

ISBN 0-7872-8717-2

Kendall/Hunt Publishing Company has the exclusive rights to reproduce this work,
to prepare derivative works from this work, to publicly distribute this work,
to publicly perform this work and to publicly display this work.

All rights reserved. No part of this publication may be reproduced,
stored in a retrieval system, or transmitted, in any form or by any
means, electronic, mechanical, photocopying, recording, or otherwise,
without the prior written permission of Kendall/Hunt Publishing Company.

Printed in the United States of America
10 9 8 7 6 5 4 3 2 1

PREFACE

The Hospice and Palliative Nurses Association is pleased to present the fourth in a series of monographs, *TREATMENT OF END-STAGE NON-CANCER DIAGNOSES,* designed to establish interdisciplinary hospice and palliative care practice guidelines for nurses in all settings.

The authors have conducted an extensive literature review and experts in the field have provided critical peer review, thus assuring a state-of-the-art practice standard.

This monograph is intended to be a living document, useful in everyday practice. Each section describes the disease process and the resulting symptoms patients will likely experience, and concludes with a useful table of possible interventions.

DISCLAIMER

HPNA will not be held liable or responsible for individual treatments, specific plans of care, or patient and family outcomes. This monograph is intended for professional educational purposes only.

Hospice and Palliative Care Clinical Practice Monograph

Treatment of End-Stage Non-Cancer Diagnoses

Shirley Ann Smith, RN, MSN, CHPN
Hospice Education Consultant
Dallas, PA

CONTRIBUTING AUTHORS

Lynn D. Borstelmann, RN, MN, CHPN, AOCN
Director, Continuum of Care Department
SUNY Upstate Medical University Hospital
Syracuse, NY

Patrick Coyne, RN, MSN, CS, CHPN
Clinical Nurse Specialist
Medical College of Virginia Hospitals
Virginia Commonwealth University
Richmond, VA

Constance M. Dahlin, RNCS, MSN, CHPN
Advanced Practice Nurse
Palliative Care Service
Massachusetts General Hospital
Boston, MA

Sheila Duffy, RN, BSN
Staff Nurse
Massachusetts General Hospital
Boston, MA

Jean Fahey, RN, MSN, CCRN, CNRN
Neuroscience Clinical Nurse Specialist
Massachusetts General Hospital
Boston, MA

Jayne Galley-Reilley, RN, BSN
Staff Nurse
Massachusetts General Hospital
Boston, MA

Nina N. Grenon, RN, CS
Adult/Geriatric Nurse Practitioner
Massachusetts General Hospital Cancer Center
Boston, MA

Debra Heidrich, RN, MSN, CHPN, AOCN
Hospice Nursing Consultant and Educator
West Chester, OH

Noreen M. Leahy, MS, RN, CS
Neuro-Oncology Nurse Practitioner
Massachusetts General Hospital
Boston, MA

Maureen Lynch, RN, MS, CS, AOPN, CHPN
Nurse Practitioner, Pain &
Symptom Management Service
Dana Farber Cancer Institute
Boston, MA

Susan B. Meyer, RN, MSN, CS, ANP
Nurse Practitioner
Transplant Unit
Norwell, MA

Kathleen Neill, RN, CS, ANP, MA, MSN
Nurse Researcher
HIV Vaccine Trials Unit
Harvard Medical School
Boston, MA

Dorothy Noyes, RN, CS
Cardiac Step-down Unit Clinical Specialist
Massachusetts General Hospital
Boston, MA

Marybeth Singer, RN, MS, CS, AOCN
Nurse Practitioner Coordinator
Hematology/Oncology
New England Medical Center
Boston, MA

Sally J. Smith, RN, MSN, CHPN
Community Health & Counseling Service
Hospice and Homecare
Elsworth, ME

Shirley Ann Smith, RN, MSN, CHPN
Hospice Education Consultant
Dallas, PA

Debra Whitaker, RN, BSN
Staff Nurse
Massachusetts General Hospital
Boston, MA

EXPERT REVIEWERS

Clare M. Conner, RN, MSN, CS
Assistant Professor
University of Vermont School of Nursing
Burlington, VT

Constance M. Dahlin, RNCS, MSN, CHPN
Advanced Practice Nurse, Palliative Care Service
Massachusetts General Hospital
Boston, MA

Pamela Fordham, RN, DSN, FNL-C
Assistant Professor of Nursing
University of Alabama at Birmingham
Birmingham, AL

Jeffrey Fudin, R. Ph., B.S., Pharm.D., DAAPM
Clinical Pharmacy Specialist in Pain Management,
VAMC—Albany, NY
Adjunct Associate Professor of Pharmacy Practice,
Albany College of Pharmacy
Adjunct Instructor of Advanced Pharmacology &
Psycho Pharmacology, SAGE Graduate School of Nursing

Linda Gorman, RN, MN, CS, OCN, CHPN
Clinical Nurse Specialist—Hospice Program
Cedars-Sinai Medical Center
Los Angeles, CA

Julie Griffie, RN, MSN, CS, AOCN
Palliative Care Advanced Practice Nurse
Medical College of Wisconsin
Milwaukee, WI

Linda King, MD
School of Medicine
Department of Medicine
Division of General Internal Medicine and Palliative Care
Shadyside Hospital
University of Pittsburgh
Pittsburgh, PA

Margaret Kush, M.D.
Clinical Instructor
Internal Medicine and Geriatrics
The Western Pennsylvania Hospital
Pittsburgh, PA

Judy Lentz, RN, MSN, OCN, NHA
Executive Director
Hospice and Palliative Nurses Association
Pittsburgh, PA

CONTENTS

I.	**Introduction**	1
II.	**Sections**	7
	General Signs and Symptoms of Dying	9
	Pulmonary Disease	21
	Heart Failure	31
	Renal Disease	37
	Liver Disease	43
	Neurological Disease	53
	Dementia	63
	Head Trauma	67
	HIV/AIDS	75
	Diabetes	83
III.	**References**	91

I

INTRODUCTION

Introduction

By Constance Dahlin and Shirley Smith

Purpose of Monograph

The mission of HPNA is to promote excellence in hospice and palliative nursing. This is partially achieved by promoting the highest professional standards of hospice and palliative nursing; and studying, researching and exchanging information, experience and ideas leading to improved nursing practice. To that end, HPNA has produced a series of four clinical monographs.

The goal of these monographs is to assist the practicing nurse in the treatment of difficult symptoms. Each monograph focuses on defining the problem, reviewing etiology and providing both pharmacological and non-pharmacological interventions. They are written by hospice and palliative nurses and reviewed by experts. The result is state of the art treatment options.

The first three monographs focused on the problematic areas that hospice and palliative care nurses frequently encounter in cancer care. They are dyspnea, terminal agitation, and nausea and vomiting. (Kuebler, 1996; Kuebler, 1997; Sheldon, 1999) They were specifically directed at the hospice nurse working within an interdisciplinary team.

This fourth monograph is of a broader scope. It is intended to provide clinical information in the more encompassing definition of palliative care. The Task Force on Palliative Care (1998) defines palliative care, as the following:

"Palliative Care refers to the comprehensive management of the physical, psychological, social, spiritual, and existential needs of patients. It is especially suited to the care of people with incurable, progressive illnesses. Palliative care affirms life and regards dying as a natural experience that is a profoundly personal experience for the individual and family. The goal of palliative care is to achieve the best possible quality of life through relief of suffering, control of symptoms and restoration of functional capacity while remaining sensitive to personal, cultural and religious values, beliefs and practices." (Task Force on Palliative Care, 1998)

Contents of Monograph

Thus, to support end of life beyond hospice and cancer care, this monograph will look at the dying process of diseases other than cancer. Its goal, in modeling the broad definition of palliative care, is to be a resource for nurses facing end of life issues in a variety of settings. This includes home care, hospice, palliative care services, acute care settings, rehabilitation settings, and nursing homes. In addition, the topics include problematic diseases that are seen in acute care such as trauma or strokes, or diseases seen in rehabilitation settings such as neurogenerative diseases, or dementia as seen in the nursing home.

There are nine non-cancer diagnoses that are examined. These diagnoses are: dementia such as Alzheimer's disease; neurodegenerative diseases such as amyotrophic lateral sclerosis, multiple sclerosis, and Parkinson's disease; cardiovascular disease such as chronic heart failure and cerebral vascular accident; respiratory disease, which includes both restrictive and obstructive diseases; AIDS; renal failure; liver diseases, such as hepatitis B, hepatitis C and cirrhosis; diabetes mellitus; and head injuries. The first eight diagnoses are commonly addressed in the literature. The last section on head trauma is addressed less frequently, though many patients die of complications of trauma.

Applying Contents to Practice

Understanding disease processes and end-stage complications is the first step in administering palliative care. The second step, of equal importance, is understanding the difference in *goals* between curative care and palliative care. In curative care, the focus is on the disease and steps to eradicate or slow down the illness trajectory. In palliative care the focus is on the person or patient/family unit and steps to ease distresses or attain specific personal goals that will optimize quality of life as defined by the patient. In practice, this means that instead of a clinician making an assessment and planning the intervention in the usual fashion, we would ascertain patient/family perceptions of the intensity of symptoms, and assess their values and goals related to proposed interventions.

In most chronic diseases, there are no cures, rather, many interventions to keep the disease under control. Since many of these diseases can continue across the lifespan, there are infinite levels of change and decline. Ideally, at the onset of those diagnoses such as cancer, renal failure, AIDS, both disease focused care and palliative care would be instituted, with the disease control having a primary role and palliative care or easing of distressing symptoms having a lesser role. Over time, as disease treatments fail or begin to produce more burden than benefit, its use would decrease and palliative/comfort care would increase. In end-stage disease, palliative care is the primary approach.

Patients may experience drug toxicities due to altered metabolism of various medications. Additionally, a patient may have a reduced response to certain medications due to decreased absorption from various administration sites (i.e. oral, subcutaneous, transdermal, sublingual, buccal, rectal).

Outcome Goals of Palliative Care

The National Hospice and Palliative Care Organization (1997) suggests three outcome goals for palliative care in terminal illness: self-determined life closure, safe and comfortable dying, and effective grieving. To accomplish these three goals for our patients, it is important to assess their values and priorities, and involve them and their families in the decision-making process.

SELF-DETERMINED LIFE CLOSURE. Self-determination means that mentally competent adult patients will have full autonomy to make decisions about how the remainder of their lives will be spent. In order to make informed decisions, the patient will need sufficient knowledge of the disease, prognosis and probable outcomes of potential interventions.

SAFE AND COMFORTABLE DYING. This goal involves treating and preventing pain and other distressing symptoms in tune with the patient's values and wishes; tailored to the patient/family functional capacity. This goal requires the involvement of an interdisciplinary team to address physical, social, spiritual, or environmental distresses and minimize crises. No treatment is given with the intention of either prolonging life or hastening death.

EFFECTIVE GRIEVING. Grief is a normal reaction to loss; its function is to enable a person's adjustment to life without the deceased and to invest in other activities and relationships. Part of palliative care is to assist patients and families through normal grieving that results in effective coping.

This monograph is intended for use in any setting where patients seek care for an incurable condition, particularly in the end stage of the disease process. All suggested interventions made in this text are compiled from palliative care experts in various settings. (Kaye, 1997; Smith, 2000; Kemp, 1999; Sheehan & Forman, 1996; Woodruff, 1999; Doyle, et al., 1998; Ferrell & Coyle, 2001). As it is read, one may find that a suggestion or treatment may be too aggressive or not aggressive enough, depending on the facility's standards of care or an individual patient's preference. It is important in each individual case to determine the value of an intervention as it relates to the goal of the intervention, the probability of it benefiting a particular patient, and the potential outcome being congruent with the patient's values.

HPNA hopes these monographs are helpful to nurses in all practice settings. If there are other areas that need to be addressed, please let us know. We strive to provide useful and pertinent information to promote excellence in end of life nursing care.

II

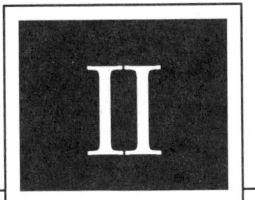

SECTIONS

General Signs and Symptoms of Dying

By Maureen Lynch

Overview

In the early 1900s, William Osler wrote that for the great majority death was a sleep and a forgetting. (Ingham, 1998) The bardo of dying from the ancient *Tibetan Book of Living and Dying* portrays dying as a less gentle process and correlates with modern descriptions of the process of dying. (Rinpoche, 1992) In the final days to hours before death, the shutting down of normal physiological processes produces a range of signs and symptoms. The signs and symptoms may vary depending on the underlying disease, specific cause of dying, and side effects of medications or other interventions in use.

In recent years, as the majority of people in the United States die in hospitals or nursing homes, we are somewhat removed from observing the natural process of dying. Therefore, patients, family members and significant others may feel overwhelmed during this time unless they have emotional support and guidance from experts in end of life care. This support can be shown in several ways (Smith, 2000):

- Acknowledge obvious signs and symptoms and explain how these are part of the normal dying process.
- Explain to loved ones that the physical, emotional, mental and spiritual dimensions may not decline simultaneously.
- Suggest ways the family members can provide comfort measures.
- Spend unhurried time just being present with patient and family members.
- Anticipate, and be prepared to respond to, intense grief reactions; the certainty of death may become real for the first time as the signs of imminent death ("active dying") are evident.
- Speak directly to the patient even when he or she is not able to respond; it shows respect for the person, and demonstrates the belief that the person may be hearing even when they cannot answer.

Common signs and symptoms seen as the body goes through the natural process of shutting down are described below.

Signs and Symptoms of Imminent Death

Mental and Spiritual Phenomenon

The dying person may sleep more of the time. This is thought to be associated with decreasing cerebral perfusion and metabolic changes. However, 6–30% of dying patients are conscious up to the time of death. (Twycross & Lichter, 1998) Disorientation to time, place and person may occur at least transiently. Decreased oxygenation and metabolic impairments may cause agitation and restlessness with or without purposeless movements. Pain, dyspnea, urinary retention and constipation may contribute to restlessness.

Reports of vision-like experiences in which the person may converse with deceased family members or friends are common. (Long, 1996; Durham & Weiss, 1997) Patients are known to use phrases like "going home" or "catching the train." They sometimes pick at blankets or sheets, or remove their clothing. Interaction with other people and the environment may be minimal with only direct auditory and tactile stimulation bringing a response. Terminal anguish marked by profound restlessness, agitation, moaning and calling out may result from emotional turmoil of unresolved conflicts, unfinished tasks, or regrets. (Twycross & Lichter, 1998) Out of character requests, gestures, or communication may mark attempts to resolve such conflicts, or a readiness to die. (Long, 1996)

The Senses

In the last days or hours, in addition to a decline in personal interactions, the senses decline as well; sight, hearing, touch, smell and taste. Vision may be increasingly diminished by loss of pupil response to light resulting finally in a fixed gaze. Pain may be associated with dying; perhaps associated with worsening pathophysiology, changes in analgesic metabolism as death approaches, or symptomatic of chronic under-treatment of pain. (Ingham, 1998) The sensation of pain may be expressed by moaning or restlessness. Hearing is thought to be the last sense to fail, so it is important to talk to the patient, convey calm reassurance and any special messages thought to be important for the patient to know.

Physical Appearance

When renal and hepatic failure occur, the body and brain are unable to cope with the resulting sequelae such as hypoxia, electrolyte imbalance, and toxin buildup related to, but not necessarily the result of, renal and/or hepatic failure. (Enck, 1994) The loss of muscle tone and body energy results in many objective physical changes. The earlobes may relax and fall back toward the head. The lower jaw may relax and the mouth falls open. The skin may be pale, blue, or gray, and cool to the touch unless the patient has a fever. The lips and fingernail beds will be very blue. Fat pads that shape the eye sockets and temples are lost to dehydration and weight loss, causing a hollowed sunken appearance of the eyes and cheeks. The nose and chin may appear pointed. Eventually multisystem failure occurs and death is imminent.

Cardiopulmonary Signs

Failing cardiac contractions cause low blood pressure, an increasingly weak and irregular pulse, and poor tissue perfusion marked by cool, mottled extremities. Increasing venous congestion creates pulmonary and hepatic congestion. Pulmonary congestion causes dyspnea, and failing neurological controls cause Cheyne-Stokes respirations marked by periods of irregular rapid shallow breaths punctuated by periods of apnea. Expiratory grunting is common. Inability to clear secretions creates the noisy respirations of the "death rattle." It is caused by the inability of the patient to expectorate pharyngeal and pulmonary secretions secondary to loss of muscle tone and reflexes. Most patients with "death rattle" are no longer aware of their surroundings, so are not suffering as a result of this. However, it is usually very stressful to relatives and significant others.

Gastrointestinal Symptoms

Dysphagia is a common symptom in the end-stages of many diseases. (Enck, 1994; Stuart, et al., 1996) This is most probably due to muscle weakness and loss of gag and swallowing reflexes. The motility and normal peristalsis of the entire gastrointestinal tract is greatly diminished by a combination of factors, including decreased physical activity, minimal intake, and opioids and other medications. This results in malabsorption, constipation and nausea. The patient may also experience indigestion, flatus, and diarrhea. The abdomen may become distended.

Hiccups sometimes occur with a distressing degree of intensity and duration. They may be self-limiting (several minutes to two days), persistent or chronic (up to one month), or intractable (lasting longer than one month). Intractable hiccups have over 100 different causes, but most often are structural, metabolic, inflammatory, or infectious disorders affecting the peripheral branches of the phrenic and/or vagus nerves. (Dahlin & Goldsmith, 2001)

Altered Metabolism

In a terminal state, it becomes evident not only that the patient has less interest in eating or drinking, but that proper absorption and metabolism does not occur. This means that the patient will not benefit from forced feeding or artificially provided feedings. The patient rarely complains of hunger or thirst and most are comfortable in a dehydrated state. (Smith, 1997) If the patient complains of thirst, or is thought to be suffering from opioid toxicity, and cannot swallow, administration of fluids (intravenously/subcutaneously) has been recommended as a manageable method in the home. (Fainsinger, et al., 1992)

Because of altered metabolism, artificially provided nutrition or hydration can produce distressful side effects such as lung congestion, edema, and nausea. The palliative approach would be to allow the patient to have whatever they want whenever they want it. Even if they have been on restricted diets in the past, at this stage they rarely eat enough to influence disease processes. So, a palliative diet order is usually "Diet as desired and tolerated." Thirst or dry mouth can be comforted by good mouth care and ice chips or sips of water, and gives families a caring role.

Social and Emotional Status

At the end of life, it is common for the dying person to become more introspective and less interested in what is happening in their surroundings. (Smith, 2000) Energy or interest in discussing business affairs or family matters may diminish. On the other hand, situations have been observed where patients seem to will themselves to resist dying until a certain event or the arrival of a certain person occurs.

The dying patient may be distressed over loss of control or function. They may have fear of the unknown about dying or an afterlife. Other emotions experienced are anger, frustration and guilt. Grief, previously known as "reactive depression" is common and is a normal response to impending death, pain, or other suffering. It is important to understand the difference between grief, depression and more serious disturbances. The American College of Physicians-American Society of Internal Medicine End of Life Consensus Panel suggests clinicians should be assuring patients that reactive distress is normal. Indeed, distress is correlated with poor quality of life and can cause much suffering. However, they note that psychological distress is under-recognized and under-treated. (Block, 2000) Clinicians should not ignore normal reactive distress or try to talk the patient into a different mind set. Rather, clinicians should acknowledge the distress, be present for tears and verbalization, and prescribe antidepressant medication if appropriate. Assisting the patient and family to explore concerns about death and dying, and the effects of illness on family, and to evaluate their strengths and resources can enhance coping and diminish distress. Patients who exhibit persistent overriding hopelessness, loss of self worth, suicidal ideation, or mood symptoms incongruent with the disease outlook are probably among the small proportion of terminal patients who may be experiencing a major depression.

Determining Prognosis in Non-Cancer Diagnoses

Although the signs and symptoms of imminent death are well defined, those signs and symptoms that mark the transition from living with a progressive life threatening illness to dying of that illness are less articulated. (Finucane, 1999) Emanuel and Emanuel (1998) suggest that preparation for a "good death" begins in the weeks and months before the actual death. During this time symptom management and interaction with patients and family can impact well being, and set the stage for peaceful death. Knowledge of prognosis impacts decisions about advanced care planning, including selection of surrogate decision makers and do not resuscitate orders, undergoing potentially curative and/or experimental therapies, futility of treatment, withholding and withdrawing treatment, and timely referral to palliative or hospice programs. (Christakis & Iwashyna, 1998; Lynn, Teno, & Harrell, 1995) Most adults indicate that if they had less than one year to live that they would want to have a realistic estimate of their expected life span. (Knaus, et al., 1995)

However, predictions about when death will occur are complex and challenging to formulate. Providers may be either overly pessimistic or optimistic in judging survival of gravely ill patients. (Lynn, Teno, & Harrell, 1995) Many feel that patients and regulatory agencies have unrealistic expectations regarding the accuracy of such predictions. (Christakis & Iwashyna, 1998) Avoidance of prognostication and discussion of the implications of prognoses with patients and families may leave patients feeling abandoned and uncertain, and the provider feeling estranged. (Knaus, et al., 1995)

Various formulas and models that can assist the clinician in formulating predictions of survival or death are reported in the literature. Most prognostic models have been developed in the oncology population where the course of illness is more defined. (Tamburini, Brumelli, Rosso, & Venafridda, 1996; Morita, Tsunda, Inoue, & Chihara, 1999; Pirovano, et al., 1999) Prediction of six month survival in patients with non-cancer diagnoses like COPD, CHF, end stage liver disease, dementia and ALS is more difficult. These conditions carry an overall poor prognosis, but patients may survive well beyond the expected period of time. (Fox, et al., 1999)

The SUPPORT (Study to Understand Prognoses and Preferences for Outcomes and Risks of Treatment) study theorized that accurate prediction of risk of death would assist clinical decision making and enhance communication regarding prognosis and preferences for treatment. The study included hospitalized patients with cancer and non-cancer diagnoses. To predict the expected 180-day survival rate of 50% in seriously ill hospitalized patients, SUPPORT utilized a computerized prognostic index. Data included age, number of days of current hospitalization, co-morbidity of cancer, major disease class, and physiological parameters (low leukocyte count, serum albumin, sodium, bilirubin, creatinine, temperature, heart rate, blood pressure, respiratory rate, oxygenation, and a coma scale). (Lynn, Teno, & Harrell, 1995; Knaus, et al., 1995; SUPPORT principle investigators, 1995) The physiological parameters were found to be most prognostic of death with the coma scale being most important of the studied physiological parameters. The computer model was at least as accurate as physician estimates of survival, and combining the prognosis derived from the computer with that of the physician enhanced accuracy. (Knaus, et al., 1995; Lynn, Teno, & Harrell, 1995)

In the SUPPORT prognostic model, certain physiological factors were more important in particular disease states. Low serum albumin was of substantial prognostic importance in patients with colon and lung cancer, and moderate importance in patients with CHF and COPD, but of relatively unimportance in coma, respiratory failure, and multiple organ system failure. Low leukocyte counts correlated more highly with poor prognosis in patients with respiratory failure and sepsis than other disease states. (Knaus, et al., 1995)

The National Hospice Organization (NHO) monograph, *Medical Guidelines for Determining Prognosis in Selected Non-Cancer Diseases* (Stuart, et al., 1996), was developed by the consensus of experts after review of available literature. (Figure 1) The NHO monograph gives specific end-stage parameters for heart disease, pulmonary, renal and liver disease, dementia, HIV, stroke and coma, and amyotrophic lateral sclerosis (ALS). In addition, there are general guidelines gleaned from the literature to suggest limited prognosis regardless of diagnosis, or in the absence of a known life-threatening diagnosis. They were intended to be a guide to aid clinicians in establishing prognoses and appropriateness for hospice. The authors advise that the key to appropriate use of the guidelines is the clinical judgement of a health care professional who can assess changes in patient's status over time, assure the patient/family's understanding of the "life-limiting" nature of the condition, and determine the patient's ideas about quality of life and goals of care. The fiscal intermediaries for Medicare now use the guidelines to help adjudge appropriate admissions by hospice programs, even though research validation has not been widely established. (Fox, Landrum-McNiff, Zhong, Dawson, Wu, & Lynn, 1999)

A study by Fox, Landrum-McNiff, Zhong, Dawson, Wu, & Lynn (1999), examined the applicability of the SUPPORT and NHO prognostic models in hospitalized patients with CHF, COPD, and ESLD (end stage liver disease). The study concluded that because deaths in these patients are often the result of sudden, unpredictable complications like infection, cardiac events, or metabolic catastrophes the models were ineffective in predicting death in the study population. The study raises several questions: Would the models have more success in determining prognosis in patients not already hospitalized? Are clinicians who know the patient able to discern prognostic clues not used in the models?

Determining what marks the transition from living with to dying as the result of an illness is complex. Assessment to establish prognosis includes the physiological parameters that mark disease progression over time and the current disease state, changes in performance or functional status, declining nutritional reserves, increasing symptom burden, fre-

FIGURE 1	General Guidelines for Limited Prognosis and Appropriateness for Palliative Care

The patient should meet the following three criteria:

I. Patient's condition is life limiting as defined by specific diagnosis, combination of diseases, or non-specific symptoms, and patient and/or family are aware of this determination.

II. Patient or family elect treatment directed toward relief of symptoms, rather than cure of underlying condition.

III. Patient has EITHER clinical progression of disease or recent impaired nutritional status:

   A. Documented clinical progression of disease, which may include:
   - Progression of disease state as documented by serial physical assessment, laboratory, radiological, or other studies.
   - Multiple emergency department visits or hospitalizations over prior six months.
   - In the absence of studies or hospital visits, clinical progression of disease may be documented by recent decline in functional status: A Karnofsky Performance Status Score ≤ 50%; or dependence in at least 3 of 6 activities of daily living (bathing, dressing, feeding, transfers, continence of urine and stool, independent ambulation to bathroom).

   B. Documented recent impaired nutritional status related to terminal process:
   - Unintentional progressive weight loss of >10% over past six months.
   - Serum albumin < 2.5 gm/dl. may be a helpful prognostic indicator but should not be used in isolation from other factors in I-III above.

Stuart, et al., 1996

quency of hospitalizations and/or emergency room visits, and the number and severity of existing medical complications. The psychological state of the patient and family is also part of the assessment. Symptoms of refractory depression such as feelings of worthlessness, hopelessness, helplessness, guilt, anhedonia, and suicidal ideation correlate with functional decline and higher mortality (von Guten & Twaddle, 1996). The patient's will to live, and self-assessment of degree of illness and quality of life are equally important.

There are indications in the literature that poor quality of life can negatively impact survival. (Addington-Hall, et al., 1990; Coates, 1997) Although quality of life is often narrowly defined as functional status, it goes beyond physical and cognitive abilities. Ferrell (1995) describes a model of quality of life that consists of physical, psychological, social and spiritual well being. The patient's sense of satisfaction in the sum of all four domains defines quality of life.

While predictive formulas and models may provide a systematic approach to some components of prognostic assessment, clinician experience, and insight into patient's individual circumstances are key to estimating the likelihood of the patient's survival or death in a specified time period. Regardless of prognosis, any patient with an incurable, progressive illness should have palliative management of distressing symptoms. Management of symptoms generally seen in end-stage diseases is seen in Table 1.

TABLE 1 — Symptom Management of General Symptoms of Dying

Symptom	Non-Prescriptive	Prescriptive
Psychological Stress, Grief, or Depression	■ Evaluate for optimal management of pain & other distressing symptoms. ■ Acknowledge feelings; "You seem depressed" or "How are your spirits today?" ■ Encourage patient to verbalize what they are feeling, without judgment or interpretation. ■ Encourage life-review; talking about the past helps the patient acknowledge satisfactions and regrets. ■ Offer relaxation exercises or relaxing activities such as music, massage or whirlpool. ■ Spend unhurried time with patient whether they wish to talk or not; mere presence is therapeutic. ■ Encourage setting of priorities and achievable goals; serves to lessen sense of hopelessness and powerlessness. ■ Assure patient that they will not be abandoned and all symptoms will receive attention.	■ Some patients can be managed with emotional support, an anxiolytic during the day and a hypnotic at night. ■ Psychostimulants help for brief periods. ■ Others may need the addition of an antidepressant: —If patient has psychomotor slowing, a less sedating drug such as fluoxetine (Prozac) might be tried. —If patient has problems related to intestinal motility or urinary retention, a drug with less anticholinergic effect, such as an SSRI (i.e. fluoxetine or paroxetine) should be used. —Most tricyclic antidepressants are started at a dose of 10–25 mg HS and gradually increased over several weeks. —The selective serotonin re-uptake inhibitors (SSRIs) such as fluoxetine (Prozac), paroxetine (Paxil) or sertraline (Zoloft), have little sedative, anticholinergic or cardiac side effects, but can cause transient anxiety, insomnia, nausea and diarrhea in the first weeks of treatment.
Terminal Secretions ("death rattle")	■ Position changes; a side/recumbent position usually decreases this symptom. ■ Suctioning has limited use; rarely a comfort measure for the patient. If necessary for the comfort of family or others, gently suction upper pharyngeal area briefly. ■ Remind family that patient is almost always oblivious to this. ■ Moisten mouth frequently if patient is mouth breathing or if anticholinergics are being used.	■ Anticholinergic drugs that suppress production of secretions. —scopolamine (0.3–0.6 mg) IM, SQ q4h or by SQ infusion or patch. —atropine (1–2 mg) IM, IV or SQ q4–6hr. —hyoscyamine, 0.125 mg SL tid to qid.
Agitation/ Delirium	■ Speak in gentle tones to the patient, explaining all events. ■ Offer family explanations of causes and stress importance of ongoing patient orientation. ■ Explain to family that it is not unusual for symptoms to exacerbate as night approaches. ■ Maintain a calm, familiar environment with minimal stimuli. ■ Offer quiet music, water fountain or "white noise" if appropriate.	■ On a trial basis, stop drugs that may be causing symptoms. ■ Hydroxyzine (Atarax, Vistaril) or lorazepam (Ativan) in low doses for mild agitation and anxiety. ■ Lorazepam or haloperidol for acute agitation and/or confusion. ■ Diazepam (Valium) is effective for agitation without psychosis or hallucinations. ■ Tricyclic antidepressants for agitated depression.

(continued)

General Signs and Symptoms of Dying

Symptom	Non-Prescriptive	Prescriptive
Spiritual Pain	■ Offer presence as a comfort and an opportunity for communication; never imposing judgment or personal beliefs. ■ Arrange clergy visits as desired by patient. ■ Listen to stories or life reviews; a good way to validate the person's value to self or others. ■ Allow expressions of anger, guilt, hurt, and fear without minimizing or explaining away. ■ Provide prayers, meditation or music as desired by the patient. ■ Encourage appropriate joy or humor; it lifts the spirit and celebrates life. ■ Determine if special rituals or observances need to be honored.	■ Address all physical distresses to free the patient for spiritual concerns; i.e., a patient in pain or nauseous cannot concentrate on anything else. ■ Never impose own beliefs or rituals.
General Concerns	■ Assist the patient in reframing goals so that they are attainable and meaningful. ■ Ascertain if there are family/social concerns that need to be addressed. ■ Show a caring attitude and openness to feelings and concerns; this enhances the potential for inner healing. ■ Create ways to give patient control; i.e., choice of food, environment, activities, etc.	■ Assure that all physical distresses are ameliorated to permit directing energies toward existential or social suffering. ■ Anxiolytics or antidepressants may be indicated.
Physical Pain	■ Assess for location, character (listen for descriptor words), duration and severity or intensity of pain (use a consistent scale to determine baseline, desired level, and effectiveness of analgesia). ■ If pain is persistent (chronic), around-the-clock (ATC) medication should be prescribed. ■ A PRN dose should be ordered in addition to ATC dosing for break-through or episodic pain. ■ If the pain is not satisfactorily relieved, some change should be made to dosage, choice of drug, adjuvants, drug therapy, psychosocial/spiritual therapies, or other areas. ■ If the pain is satisfactorily relieved by the current dosing, but consistently recurs before the next dose, the interval needs to be shortened. ■ Adjuvant drugs may be those that relieve other symptoms that may be exacerbating the perception of pain, or those that have a specific analgesic action. ■ Massage, whirlpool, distraction, etc.	■ Pain intensity should be matched to analgesic strength: —for mild pain: use mild analgesia; use non-opioids such as acetaminophen, NSAIDS. —for moderate pain: use mild opioids, such as codeine. —for severe pain, use opioids such as morphine or equivalents. ■ Adjuvant medications may include steroids, antianxiety agents, muscle relaxants, or butyrophenones (Haloperidol), etc. ■ Tricyclic antidepressants and anticonvulsants have specific action to relieve neuropathic pains. ■ Avoid drugs that have short duration, too many side effects or otherwise not appropriate for good pain management: meperidine (Demerol), dronabinol (Marinol), pentazocine (Talwin), butorphanol (Stadol), nalbuphine (Nubain), ketorolac (Toradol), or placebos. ■ Prophylactic bowel regime should be initiated for patients on ATC opioids.

(continued)

Symptom	Non-Prescriptive	Prescriptive
Cough	■ Assess for precipitating factors such as dry air, cool drafts, or cigarette smoke. ■ Note relationship to intake, such as milk products, cold liquids, etc. ■ Offer warm drinks or cough drops. ■ Humidify room air if dryness is a problem.	■ Expectorants and mucolytics (terpin hydrate or guaifenesin) for productive cough. ■ Codeine 5–30 mg q4h PRN (dose depends on severity and whether patient is already on opioids), or: ■ Morphine sulfate 2–10 mg PO q4h PRN (regulate as for codeine). ■ Terminal phase coughing can be relieved with atropine or scopolamine. ■ Treat contributing causes as reasonable: COPD, CHF, infections, or GERD.
Anxiety, insomnia, restlessness	■ Assess for pain, fear, or air hunger. ■ Talk with, listen to, walk with, or sit by the patient. ■ Ask volunteers or loved ones to be present with patient if this is comforting to the patient. ■ Decrease stimulation and demands. ■ Suggest tub baths, backrubs or other relaxation methods. ■ Change environment according to patient needs (e.g., leave lights on, allow patient to sleep in a lounge chair). ■ Discuss with patient/family if night insomnia is a problem; medication is not necessary if being awake at night is not distressing to anyone involved; most seriously ill patients do not have normal sleep patterns.	■ For anxiety/restlessness: —lorazepam (Ativan) 0.5–2 mg PO QID; or —diazepam (Valium) 2–10 mg PO, IM or SL, TID or QID. ■ For insomnia: Same doses as above at bedtime; or —diphenhydramine (Benadryl) 25–50 mg PO at bedtime; or —amitriptyline (Elavil) 25–150 mg nightly 1–2 hours before bedtime.
Dyspnea	■ Plan care and activities to decrease exertional dyspnea. ■ Position the patient for comfort, sitting upright in bed or chair and/or with arms propped up over pillows on a table in front of patient. ■ Provide calming and reassurance through the presence of a supportive person. ■ Encourage relaxation by using a gentle voice, gentle touching, and guiding slow, deep breaths. ■ Keep room cool and control humidity, depending on patient preferences. ■ Move air in room by fan or by opening window. ■ Solicit patient fears and give reassurance about the availability of medications and team members.	■ Morphine sulfate (MS), 5–20 mg SC or 15–60 mg PO q3h PRN; may repeat in 3 hours if needed. MS reduces inappropriate tachypnea and overventilation of the large airways, making breathing more efficient and without carbon dioxide retention. For the opioid-naïve patient, begin with 2.5 mg SC (7.5 mg PO) dose. ■ Anxiolytics, such as lorazepam (Ativan) 0.5–2 mg q4–6h PRN, can be added to address the anxiety component in dyspnea. Diazepam (Valium) 5–10 mg IM or PO q6h PRN is effective, but has a longer half-life. ■ Bronchodilators, nebulizers, or steroids may be added but generally are helpful only if the patient has a history of these being effective in prior obstructive airway disease.

(continued)

General Signs and Symptoms of Dying

Symptom	Non-Prescriptive	Prescriptive
Dysphagia	■ Elevate upper torso during meals and for 30 minutes afterward. ■ Tipping the chin slightly downward will decrease likelihood of aspiration. ■ Pay close attention to good oral hygiene. ■ Work with patient and family to determine the consistency of food best tolerated. Do not assume that liquids or soft foods are preferable.	■ Treat Candida oral infections with nystatin suspension or fluconazole PO. ■ Local relief of mouth or throat pain with viscous lidocaine, 2%; however, numbing effect must be evaluated before feeding (may need to time feeding an hour or so later). ■ Dexamethasone 8–12 mg/day may offer temporary relief by reducing inflammatory edema, but after a few weeks myopathy and other steroid side effects may develop. ■ More aggressive measures such as bypass surgery, laser treatment, or endoprosthetic intubation are rarely indicated in seriously ill patients due to the high probability of complications. The symptom of dysphagia itself portends limited prognosis.
Skin Breakdown, Pressure Ulcers	■ Maintain good position and body alignment. ■ Turn patient at least q2hours. ■ Keep skin dry and clean. ■ Use pressure-releasing devices such as pillows, pads and special mattresses. ■ In repositioning or transferring patient, use techniques that reduce friction or pressure. Allowing a reddened area (Stage I) to rub against sheets can cause a blister or break the skin (Stage II). ■ Encourage as much mobility as possible.	■ Stage I (redness): creams, ointments, or sprays (such as A&D or aloe). ■ Stage II (blister or break in skin): semipermeable dressing (e.g., bioclusives or hydrocolloidal dressings such as Duoderm) if no infection is present. ■ Stage III (destruction of subcutaneous tissue): surgical debridement, wet-to-dry saline dressings, hydrocolloidal dressings, antimicrobials, hydrogen peroxide, and/or whirlpool therapy. ■ Stage IV (muscle or bone involvement): wet-to-dry dressings; surgical debridement may be needed depending on disease trajectory. ■ For skin/wound infections, appropriate oral or topical antibiotics as warranted to help infection and odor.
Peripheral edema	■ Encourage exercise, especially leg exercises, even if patient is bed bound (if not distressing to terminally ill patient). ■ Leg elevation helps but only when legs are even or higher than heart level. For this reason, it is seldom useful to elevate legs while patient is sitting in a chair. ■ Encourage increase in dietary protein in cases where the patient is able and willing. ■ MLD (manual lymphatic drainage)	■ Compression stockings (thigh-high) for daytime out-of-bed hours for extreme or severe cases. ■ Cautious use of oral diuretics, such as hydrochlorothiazide (Hydrazide) in a moderate dose three times weekly as a trial; watching for patient distresses associated with diuresis and symptoms of electrolyte imbalance.

(continued)

Symptom	Non-Prescriptive	Prescriptive
Nausea, Vomiting	■ Assess the patient for relationship of nausea to particular medications, foods, or activities. ■ Allow patient to self-regulate intake, suggesting decrease in fatty, gas forming, or fried foods. ■ Eliminate strong or repulsive odors. ■ Offer small frequent meals rather than three big meals/day. ■ Activities that relax and distract patient are beneficial to treat any psychological component.	■ Discontinue offending medications when identified and if possible. ■ Always provide for PRN antiemetic when starting opioids for the first time. ■ If symptoms derive from liver failure, consider a trial of lactulose (Cephylac) 30cc TID adjusted to achieve 2–3 soft stools per day. ■ If gastric irritation is present from medication or known peptic ulcer disease, an H_2 receptor antagonist: ranitidine (Zantac) or famotidine (Pepsid) or a proton pump inhibitor such as omeprazole (Prilosec). ■ Prochlorperazine (Compazine) 10 mg PO or IM q4h PRN, or 25 mg rectally q12h PRN is a common protocol. ■ Haloperidol (Haldol), 0.5–2 mg PO or SC q6h PRN is good because it is a strong antiemetic causing low sedation; and is good for other symptoms at the same time, such as agitation or anxiety.
Anorexia, Weight Loss	■ Encourage high-protein/high-calorie foods such as eggs, milk shakes, custards, peanut butter, and cream soups. ■ Powdered nutritional supplements can be added to other foods without adding volume. ■ Do not push foods that cause a metallic or bitter taste. These are usually red meats; fish or poultry could be offered instead. ■ Provide food whenever patient expresses hunger; do not wait for "mealtimes." ■ Remove food when patient is finished. ■ Make the atmosphere and food presentation as pleasant as possible. ■ Check dentures for fit; weight loss may necessitate relining. ■ For the end-stage patient, avoid weighing, it places undue emphasis on weight loss. ■ Beer, wine or sherry before meals may help appetite. ■ Offer favorite foods; anticipate this can change as disease progresses. ■ Understand that patients may request foods and upon delivery be unable to consume.	■ Eliminate any medications when possible that may be causing nausea. ■ If nausea is a problem, there should be a standing order for antiemetic; may need to try several to find the one that works best for each individual patient. ■ Steroids may stimulate appetite; discontinue if side effects outweigh benefits. ■ Megesterol acetate (Megace) in doses of 400 mg BID may increase appetite. ■ If patient is end-stage and eating very little, they generally don't need to be on restricted diets; should have "diet as desired and tolerated." ■ Considerations for providing artificial nutrition and hydration (ANH): —prognosis: this is key because if patient is in last weeks or months, studies show that they will gradually decrease intake, are more comfortable and do not suffer from dehydration or distressful electrolyte abnormalities. —goal of treatment: any ANH should be for increased comfort, strength, or longevity; if these goals are not likely to be achieved, ANH is inappropriate. —patient's goals & values: ascertain if the patient wants to have a trial of ANH. —if patient is dehydrated & suffering from retained opioid metabolites, some will benefit from subcutaneous fluid administration.

Compiled from: Kaye 1997; Smith, 2000; Kemp, 1999; Sheehan & Forman, 1996; Woodruff, 1999; Doyle, et al., 1998; Ferrell & Coyle, 2001.

Pulmonary Disease

By Nina N. Grenon

Overview

The term chronic obstructive pulmonary disease (COPD), indicates a group of respiratory diseases characterized by chronic and recurrent obstructed airflow in the pulmonary pathways. (Porth, 1998) The disease process ranges from partially reversible abnormalities to end-stage cardiopulmonary insufficiency. The typical patient with COPD has smoked more than 20 pack/years before symptoms develop.

It is estimated that in the United States, approximately 14 million people suffer from COPD. (American Thoracic Society, 1995) There were 85,544 deaths from COPD in 1991, a death rate of 18.6 per 100,000 people; the 4th leading cause of death. When adjusted by age, the death rate from COPD rose 72% in the twenty-year period between 1966 and 1986. This is particularly important because death rates from all causes in that same period decreased 22% and the death rates from heart and cerebrovascular disease declined 45% and 85%, respectively. Observed increases in morbidity and mortality from COPD appear to be related to past trends in cigarette smoking and the increasing number of people living longer. Since smoking frequency has fallen over the past 30 years, a decrease in COPD mortality in coming decades is anticipated. (American Thoracic Society, 1995)

Pathophysiology

Multiple pathways are implicated in the development of COPD. Emphysema (type A COPD) and bronchitis (type B COPD) may be discrete diseases, but most often, patients present with some combination of these disorders, thus complicating the clinical picture. (Porth, 1998)

Obstructive Pulmonary Disease

In COPD, there is enlargement of bronchial mucous glands, dilatation of gland ducts, and structural changes of bronchi and bronchioles, including denuding of cilia on the epithelial surfaces. Hypertrophy of the bronchial mucous glands causes excessive mucous production. The mucous is thick and tenacious and ciliary activity is impaired, making mucous clearance difficult. Thus, the defense mechanisms of the bronchi are compromised, resulting in increased susceptibility to infection and pneumonia. (Eckman, et al., 1998) Infection and injury further increase mucous production. The bronchial wall becomes inflamed and thickened from edema and build-up of inflammatory cells. Eventually all airways become affected, and the bronchial smooth muscle becomes hypertrophied. The combination of hypertrophied smooth muscle and thick mucous obstructs the airway, especially during expiration, when it is already narrowed. This, in turn, leads to ventilation perfusion mismatch, hypoventilation and hypoxemia. (Porth, 1998)

EMPHYSEMA. In emphysema (type A COPD), the terminal bronchioles enlarge and the alveoli become fragmented, secondary to destruction of connective tissue by proteases (enzymes that digest proteins). These proteases, particularly elastase (an enzyme that digests elastin), are normally kept in balance by an anti-protease enzyme called alpha-1-antitrypsin (A1AT). If there are low levels of A1AT, the process of elastic tissue destruction goes unchecked. (Porth, 1998) A hereditary deficiency of A1AT accounts for about 1% of all cases of COPD and is more common in young persons with COPD. There is evidence that cigarette smoking reduces body stores of A1AT, and at the same time increases the number of macrophages and neutrophils in the alveolar walls. The presence of additional macrophages and neutrophils increases the pathology as they are the cells that release proteases. (Porth, 1998)

The pathologic changes in emphysema lead to a loss of elastic recoil and airway support, setting off a cascade of decreasing efficiency of oxygenation. Elastic recoil is lost due to destruction of elastin and collagen in the lung parenchyma, leading to over-distention of the lungs. This loss of lung parenchymal tissue causes the terminal airways to collapse or narrow, particularly during expiration. Air is then trapped in the distal air spaces, causing further distention of the lungs. As the over-distended lung presses against the diaphragm, ventilation diminishes. Then, as the patient works harder to force trapped air out of the lungs, intrapleural pressure increases, leading to more airway collapse. (Eckman, et al., 1998)

BRONCHITIS. In chronic bronchitis (type B COPD), the destruction of the alveolar and bronchiolar walls decreases the alveolar capillary membrane surface area, causing impaired gas exchange. Hypoxemia, hypercarbia, and cyanosis develop, reflecting an imbalance between ventilation and perfusion. Hypoxemia becomes a stimulus for increased vascular constriction and red cell production. (Porth, 1998) Diffusion abnormalities and airway obstruction may or may not lead to a retention of carbon dioxide. Also, pulmonary vasoconstriction reduced pulmonary diffusion. Hypoxemia, which causes generalized pulmonary artery constriction, and pressure from over-distended alveoli, further impairs diffusion capacity. A reduction in total cross-sectional area of the pulmonary vascular bed, constriction of vascular smooth muscle in pulmonary artery and arterioles, and the destruction of alveolar septa, will eventually lead to pulmonary hypertension. (Ingram, 1994) If pulmonary hypertension is prolonged, the increase on the right ventricle leads to cor pulmonale, a condition in which the right ventricle dilates, hypertrophies, or both, in an attempt to overcome increase in pulmonary pressure. Eventually, cor pulmonale in association with abnormal blood gases ultimately leads to right ventricular failure. (Eckman, 1998)

The mnemonics "pink puffer" and "blue bloater" have been used to differentiate the clinical manifestations of emphysema and chronic bronchitis. The important features of these two forms of COPD are described in Figure 2. In practice, differentiation between the two types is not as vivid as presented in the figure, as patients often have symptoms of more than one disease entity.

Restrictive Pulmonary Disease

Restrictive disorders are those in which the mobility or functioning parenchyma is decreased for some reason. Functional lung volume will be decreased by restricted movement/restricted expansion of the thoracic cage; for example, secondary to kyphoscoliosis, pleuritic pain, idio-

FIGURE 2 | Clinical Features of Type A and Type B COPD

Criteria	Type A COPD	Type B COPD
Disease entity	Emphysema predominant	Bronchitis predominant
Syndrome name	Pink puffer	Blue bloater
Appearance	Thin, wasted	Obese and/or edema 2° right ventricular failure
Major symptom	Dyspnea	Productive cough
PO_2	Normal until late stage	Low
PCO_2	Normal until late stage	Normal or elevated
Elastic recoil of lung	Decreased	Normal
Diffusing capacity	Decreased	Normal
Hematocrit	Normal	Often increased (secondary polycythemia)
Cor pulmonale	Infrequent	Common
Cyanosis	Rare	Marked
Cardiac enlargement	Minimal	Marked
Sputum production	Minimal	Marked
Lung capacity	Increased	Decreased

Compiled from Porth, 1998; Ingram, 1994; Eckman, 1998.

pathic interstitial fibrosis, muscular dystrophy or abdominal distention. Weakness and paralysis of respiratory muscles are possible complications of Guillain-Barre syndrome, myasthenia gravis, or other neuromuscular diseases and may be part of general debility of terminal illness. Space occupying lesions, pleural effusions, or tuberculosis are examples of conditions that can decrease both the mobility and the functional surface area for gas exchange.

Advanced Stage Symptoms

Both types of lung disease eventually lead to respiratory failure, i.e., the inability of the pulmonary system to adequately oxygenate body systems. Hypoxemia and hypercapnia lead to increased pulmonary pressure which will result in right ventricular failure (cor pulmonale); the patient will experience feelings of breathlessness and suffocation, limited tolerance to physical activity, and poor quality of life.

The patient will have some degree of cyanosis. There is decreased motion of the diaphragm and rib expansion. Expiration often occurs through pursed lips. Breath sounds are decreased, expiration is prolonged, and heart sounds become distant. Coarse crackles may be heard at the lung bases. The accessory muscles of the neck and shoulder are used; retraction of the supraclavicular fossae as well as contraction of the abdominal muscles will be noted on inspiration. Heart failure will result in distended neck veins, hepatomegaly and peripheral edema.

Electrolyte disturbances are common in patients with COPD. Hypophosphatemia, hyperkalemia, hypocalcemia, and hypomagnesemia are common and are associated with diminished diaphragmatic function. Correction of abnormal electrolytes, especially phosphorus, results in improved respiratory function.

Clinical data indicates that outcome following an episode of respiratory failure correlates with the severity of the underlying COPD and patient activity level while in a stable period.

(Dardes, Campo and Chiappini, 1986). Patients who have poor baseline function, marginal nutritional status, severely restricted activity, and deterioration of late stage pulmonary dysfunction, may elect to forgo intubation, if in the judgment of both patient and clinician, it would only temporarily interrupt the terminal phase of the disease. (American Thoracic Society, 1995).

Determining prognosis in end-stage lung disease requires clinical judgment as well as looking at specific factors, as it is extremely difficult to predict with accuracy. Obviously, as symptoms become more severe and acute episodes more frequent, it is clear that the disease is progressing. Another indicator is decreasing efficacy of treatments which have helped in the past. The "Medical Guidelines for Determining Prognosis in Selected Non-Cancer Diseases" published by the National Hospice and Palliative Care Organization, suggest parameters that indicate a limited prognosis in pulmonary disease:

- Hypoxemic at rest on supplemental oxygen
  - pO_2 ≤55mm Hg on supplemental O_2
  - O_2 saturation ≤88% on supplemental O_2
- Persistent symptoms of severe cough, copious sputum and recurrent infections
- Disabling dyspnea at rest; poor or unresponsive to bronchodilators
- Forced expiratory volume in one second (FEV1) after bronchodilator: <30% of predicted
- Decrease in FEV1 on serial testing of >40 ml per year
- Right heart failure due to lung disease
- Hypercapnia (pCO_2 ≥ 50 mm Hg)
- Unintentional weight loss > 10% of body weight in past six months
- Resting tachycardia (heart rate > 100 per minute)

Management of Symptoms

Sedatives and opioids are indicated to relieve severe distress, with dosages increased slowly over several days to achieve the desired effect. Tolerance to the effects of opioids and sedatives in depressing the respiratory center usually occurs more quickly than does the tolerance to the beneficial effects. In the presence of renal insufficiency, which occurs with the aging process, agents with a shorter half-life are preferred. (American Thoracic Society, 1995) Agitated ventilated patients may need sedation, for example, with haloperidol, because it calms agitation and confusion without depressing the respiratory center. (Wheeler, 1993)

Drug therapy of COPD or resulting heart failure should be utilized according to the severity of the disease and on how a patient tolerates specific drugs. (Celli, 1998) Guidelines of the most common drugs, dosages and precautions are outlined in Figures 6, 7 and 8. There is no evidence that regular use of any of these drugs alters the progression of chronic obstructive pulmonary disease. However, they may alleviate symptoms, improve activity tolerance, and improve quality of life. The major distressing symptoms observed in these patients are dyspnea, cough, acute and sudden paroxysmal attacks, insomnia, anxiety, weakness, and depression. Treatments for these symptoms are outlined in the following table.

TABLE 2	Symptom Management of Pulmonary Disease	
Symptom	Non-Prescriptive	Prescriptive
Dyspnea	■ Breathing retraining. (*See Figure 3*) ■ Position for ease of breathing: sitting upright, leaning forward with hands on knees or table. ■ Provide calming effect by reassurance and presence of supportive person. ■ Encourage relaxation by gentle voice, gentle touching and guiding slow deep breaths. ■ Keep room cool and control humidity. ■ Move air in room by fan or open window. ■ Plan care and activities to decrease exertional dyspnea.	■ Oxygen. (*See guidelines in Figures 3, 4 and 5*) ■ Morphine sulfate, 5mg SC or 10–15 mg PO or 5 mg SL q3h PRN; may repeat in 20 minutes if needed. MS reduces inappropriate tachypnea and over-ventilation of the large airways, making breathing more efficient and without CO_2 retention. For opioid-naïve patient, begin with 2.5–5 mg. dose. ■ Bronchodilators. (*See guidelines in Figures 6, 7 and 8*). Antibiotics if acute bacterial infection present. (Older agents such as tetracycline, doxycycline, amoxicillin, erythromycin, trimethoprim-sulfamethoxazole, or cefaclor are effective and less costly.) ■ Steroids. (*See guidelines in Figure 8*). ■ Anxiolytics for the anxiety element compounding the problem (Lorazepam 0.5–2 mg PO/IV/IM q8h prn).
Cough	■ Assess for environmental irritants such as dry air, drafts, cigarette smoke, offending odors. ■ Assist patient in identifying precipitating factors such as milk products, cold liquids, etc. ■ Warm drinks or cough drops. ■ Humidify room air if dryness is a problem.	■ Expectorants and mucolytics for productive cough. Codeine 5–30 mg q4h PRN or Morphine sulfate 2–10 mg q4h PRN. ■ Benzonatate (Tessalon Perles) to anesthetize respiratory stretch receptors—only in dry cough. ■ Nebulized local anesthetic (lidocaine 2%) can be used q2–6hr (NPO ×30 minutes after treatment).
Acute and Sudden Paroxysmal Attack of Dyspnea or Cough	■ Check O_2 and pulse oximeter if available.	■ Morphine sulfate 5–20 mg PO q15 minutes or 1–3 mg IV. ■ Short acting benzodiazepines can be quickly titrated to desired level of comfort; sedation may be more desirable than unrelieved dyspnea with high levels of anxiety.
Anxiety or Insomnia	■ Assess if fear, pain or air hunger is present. ■ Arrange for someone to be with patient if possible and appropriate. ■ Offer back rubs, soothing music, or guided imagery for relaxation. ■ Change environment according to patient needs, e.g., lights on, out of bed, etc. ■ Consider drug-related causes: caffeine, xanthines, corticosteroids, amphetamines, etc.	■ Anxiolytics such as lorazepam (Ativan) 0.5–2 mg PO QID; or diazepam (Valium) 2–10 mg PO, IM, SL, TID or QID. ■ For insomnia: above meds at bedtime, or diphenhydramine (Benadryl) 25–50 mg PO HS; or amitriptyline (Elavil) 25–150 mg 2 hrs before bedtime. ■ Temazepam (Restoril), 15–30 mg HS PRN.

(continued)

Symptom	Non-Prescriptive	Prescriptive
Weakness	■ Assist patient in listing priorities and planning to conserve energy for special events and desired activities. ■ Assess need for equipment to assist patient with independence and ambulating: walkers, handrails, raised toilet seat, etc. ■ Encourage nutrition and hydration to extent patient can tolerate.	■ Discontinue any unnecessary antihypertensives. ■ Evaluate for hypokalemia if patient has been on diuretics or has persistent vomiting or diarrhea. ■ Dexamethasone PO 4 mg/day may give "sense of well-being" but patient should be warned against unrealistic expectations, i.e., side effects could cause other problems.
Depression	■ Acknowledge the normalcy of reactive depression and let patient decide if treatment is warranted. ■ Encourage mental and physical activities that may add meaning and satisfaction. ■ Involve family, friends, and clergy as indicated. —Promote autonomy and control wherever possible. —Increase patient and family participation in care. —Maximize symptom management to decrease physical stress. —Assist patient to draw on sources of strength e.g., faith or other belief systems. —Refer as appropriate for those experiencing significant inability to cope. —Allow the patient to be independent whenever possible. —Answer patient's questions in an honest and sensitive manner. —Assess need for further intervention or referral to mental health.	■ Amitriptyline (Elavil) 25–150 mg PO HS. Begin with low dose and increase by 25–50 mg q2–3 days as tolerated. Amitriptyline is antidepressive/anxiolytic and mildly sedative which help sleep when taken in the evening. ■ Doxepin (Sinequan) 50–150 mg PO HS, titrated as above. ■ SSRIs, SARIs, and SNRIs have fewer side effects and may offer a better tolerated alternative.

Compiled from: Kaye, 1997; Smith, 2000; Kemp, 1999; Sheehan & Forman, 1996; Woodruff, 1999; Doyle, et al., 1998; Ferrell & Coyle, 2001.

FIGURE 3 | Breathing Retraining for Patients with COPD and Others with Dyspnea

The goal is to help the patient relieve and control breathlessness and counteract such physiologic abnormalities as hyperinflation related to chronic airflow obstruction. Retraining techniques work to:

1. Improve the ventilatory pattern (i.e., slow respiratory rate and increased tidal volume),
2. Prevent dynamic airway compression,
3. Improve respiratory synchrony of abdominal and thoracic musculature, and
4. Improve gas exchange.

Although many patients with COPD self-discover pursed lip breathing on their own, specific instruction can be given to decrease dyspnea as follows:

1. Breathe in slowly and deeply through the nose.
2. Purse the lips tightly as if to whistle.
3. Then breathe out slowly through the pursed lips, taking twice as long to exhale as to inhale.

Adapted from Celli, BR and American Thoracic Society, 1995.

| **FIGURE 4** | Summary of Guidelines for Oxygen Use from the Palliative Care Literature |

1. Oxygen therapy is of benefit to patients with documented hypoxia.
2. Significant hypoxemia can be ascertained by pulse oximeter (saturation < 90%).
3. If dyspnea is only on exertion, reserve oxygen for exacerbations and before exercise.
4. For many patients, periodic low doses of morphine, as needed for dyspnea, is as effective as oxygen administration, and avoids the confinement and drying effect of oxygen administration.
5. Oxygen therapy must be used with caution in patients with COPD and hypoxia as they depend on the hypoxia and elevated carbon dioxide for respiratory drive.
6. A portable oxygen concentrator is the easiest and most economical means of providing oxygen therapy in the home.
7. Sometimes oxygen not needed, but patients benefit from flow of air from fan.

Adapted from Woodruff, 1999; Smith 2000; Doyle, et al., 1998.

| **FIGURE 5** | Indications for Long-Term Oxygen Therapy |

Absolute

- $PaO_2 \leq 55$ mm Hg or $SaO_2 \leq 88\%$

In presence of cor pulmonale:

- PaO_2 55–59 mm Hg or $SaO_2 \leq 89\%$
- EKG evidence of "P" pulmonale, hematocrit > 55%, congestive heart failure

Only in specific situations:

- $PaO_2 \geq 60$ mm Hg or $SaO_2 \leq 90\%$
- With lung disease and other clinical needs, such as sleep apnea with nocturnal desaturation not corrected by CPAP

If the patient meets criteria at rest, O_2 should also be prescribed during sleep and exercise, appropriately titrated.

If the patient is normoxemic at rest, but desaturates during exercise or sleep ($PaO_2 \leq 55$ mm Hg), O_2 should be prescribed for these indications.

Also consider nasal CPAP or BiPAP.

The values do not have to be present to order oxygen therapy. Dyspnea is a symptom and what patient says it is. Considering a trial of oxygen therapy is warranted.

Definition of abbreviations CPAP = continuous positive airway pressure; EKG = electrocardiogram; BiPAP = bilevel positive airway pressure.

From American Thoracic Society Standards for the Diagnosis and Care of Patients with Chronic Obstructive Pulmonary Disease. (1995). American Journal of Respiratory and Critical Care Medicine, Vol. 152, No. 5, p S92. Reprinted with permission.

FIGURE 6 | Step-By-Step Pharmacologic Therapy for COPD

1. For mild, variable symptoms:
   - Selective β_2-agonist metered dose inhaler (MDI) aerosol, 1–2 puffs every 2-6 h as needed, not to exceed 8–12 puffs per 24 h
2. For mild to moderate continuing symptoms:
   - Ipratropium MDI aerosol, 2–6 puffs every 6–8 h; not to be used more frequently; plus
   - Selective β-agonist MDI aerosol (excluding salmeterol), 1–4 puffs as required four times daily for rapid relief, when needed, or as a regular supplement
3. If response to step 2 is unsatisfactory, or there is a mild to moderate increase in symptoms:
   - Add sustained release theophylline, 200–400 mg twice daily for nocturnal bronchospasm; if no improvement with blood level between 10–18 mcg/ml, discontinue theophylline.
   - Consider use of mucokinetic agent
4. If control of symptoms is suboptimal:
   - Consider course of oral steroids (e.g., prednisone), up to 40 mg/d for 10–14d
     —If improvement occurs, wean to low daily or alternate-day dose, e.g., 7.5 mg
     —If steroid appears to help, consider possible use of aerosol steroid MDI, particularly if patient has evidence of bronchial hyperreactivity
5. For severe exacerbation:
   - Increase β_2-agonist dosage, e.g., MDI with spacer 6–8 puffs every ½–2 h or subcutaneous administration of epinephrine, 0.5–1.0 mg, or terbutaline, 0.25–0.5 mg; and/or
   - Increase ipratropium dosage, e.g., MDI with spacer 6–8 puffs every 3–4 h or inhalant solution of ipratropium 0.5 mg every 4–8 h; and
   - Provide aminophylline dosage intravenously with calculated amount to bring serum theophylline level to 10–12 µg/ml; and
   - Provide methylprednisolone dosage intravenously giving 50–100 mg immediately, then every 6–8 h; and add:
     —An antibiotic, if indicated
     —A mucokinetic agent if sputum is very viscous

From American Thoracic Society Standards for the Diagnosis and Care of Patients with Chronic Obstructive Pulmonary Disease. (1995). American Journal of Respiratory and Critical Care Medicine, Vol. 152, No. 5, p S86. Reprinted with permission.

FIGURE 7 | COPD Drugs

Beta-agonists	albuterol pirbuterol metaproterenol terbutaline isoetherine	A spacer should be used to improve aerosol delivery and reduce side effects (SE). The rapid onset of action may lead patients to over use; exceeding doses may lead to cardiac arrhythmias, nausea & vomiting, tremors, etc. Should be administered with foods to decrease gastric irritation; tricyclic antidepressants, MAOIs, in addition to sympathomimetics may ↑ hyperexcitability associated with beta-agonists.
Anticholinergics	ipratropium	Limit dosing; SE as above.
Xanthines	Aminophylline/ Theophylline/caffeine	SE include: convulsions, nausea

Adapted from Celli, BR & American Thoracic Society, 1995.

| FIGURE 8 | Precautions in COPD Drug Use |

Precautions when using beta-agonists
- Watch for nonimprovement or paradoxical deterioration with aerosol use
- Use spacers to improve compliance and reduce systemic side effects
- Avoid overuse; check number of metered dose inhalers (MDIs) and puffs per MDI to monitor patient
- Instruct patient on maximum number of puffs per day, and number allowed during an exacerbation
- If a long-acting agent is used, caution patient that frequent use must be avoided
- Home updraft nebulizers with inhalant solutions that provide large dosages are rarely needed

Precautions when using theophylline:
- Initiate treatment with a low dose (e.g., 400 mg/d) and adjust after a five days, based on serum level
- Reduce dosage if drug clearance is likely to be impaired because of illness, liver malfunction, or concomitant drugs
- Do not allow any additional theophylline preparation to be taken, avoid caffeine
- Drug must be taken at the same time each day with respect to meals
- When symptoms change, acute illness develops, new drugs are added, or symptoms suggestive of toxicity develop, check serum level of theophylline
- Aim for a serum level of 8–12 µg/ml; adjust dosage and follow serum level when indicated

Precautions when using ipratropium
- Patients should generally use a spacer and should avoid spraying into eyes
- Be prepared to increase dose if necessary from 2–3 puffs 3–4 times a day to 6–8 puffs 3–4 times a day, if tolerated
- Caution patient that onset of effect is relatively slow; additional doses should not be taken for acute symptom relief
- Monitor for side effects, e.g., tachycardia, dry mouth, glaucoma, prostatism, or bladder neck obstruction

Precautions when using oral steroids
- Reduce dosage to lowest effective daily dose or to alternate-day dosing as quickly as symptoms allow. If steroid dose is being decreased due to potential for long term toxicity, consider long term prognosis of patient.
- Monitor for hypertension, diabetes, mental changes, purpura
- Distinguish psychological benefit from true pulmonary benefit by following FEV_1 for 2 wk after initiating therapy
- Steroid-dependent patients require steroid coverage during any crisis for many months after stopping steroids
- Repeatedly evaluate patient to determine if steroid therapy can be discontinued

Precautions when using aerosol steroids
- Seek objective evidence of the value of this therapy because its use may decrease compliance with other aerosol usage
- Use a spacer; monitor for oral thrush and laryngeal dysfunction
- Be aware that aerosol steroid side effects may occur in skin, bone, etc.
- When introducing aerosol steroids in a patient on an oral steroid, wean slowly off the oral drug
- Rinse mouth after each dose to reduce incidence of steroid-induced candida.

From American Thoracic Society Standards for the Diagnosis and Care of Patients with Chronic Obstructive Pulmonary Disease. (1995). American Journal of Respiratory and Critical Care Medicine, Vol. 152, No. 5, p S88. Reprinted with permission.

Heart Failure

By Dorothy Noyes

Overview

It is estimated that 400,000 new cases of heart failure (HF) are diagnosed every year and that about 1–2% of the population 65 years and older in the US are currently living with heart failure. Heart failure is not only one of the leading causes of death and disability in older people in Western countries, it is also a major cause of morbidity and contributes greatly to health care costs. (USDHHS, 1994) Predictions are for an exponential growth in the number of people living with heart failure. Improved therapies for hypertension and ischemic heart disease are allowing patients with these disorders to survive (or avoid) other clinical manifestations, only to develop HF in later life. Improvements in the treatment of myocardial infarction, hypertension, and even end-stage renal disease have all contributed to the increasing incidence of HF. (Rich, 1997)

Pathophysiology

Heart failure (HF) is the common terminal pathway for many cardiovascular diseases. HF is a condition in which the heart is unable to pump blood at the rate required by metabolizing tissues or when the heart can do so only at elevated filling pressures. (AHCPR, 1994) It is not a single disease but a symptom complex reflective of effort intolerance, fluid retention and reduced longevity. The cause may be from myocardial contractile failure (impaired contraction and emptying) due to ischemic heart disease, myocarditis, or cardiomyopathy or a disorder that prevents proper filling or emptying of the heart such as valvular regurgitation or pericardial disease. Other diseases that may result in HF are high pressure overloads like hypertension or high output overloads such as renal failure, anemia, AV fistula, sepsis, or thyrotoxicosis. High output demands cause the heart to fail because the heart's coronary flow is inadequate to address the increased metabolic needs of the overworked myocardium. (Smith & Campine, 1984)

Mortality

The diagnosis of heart failure carries a significant risk of mortality. In the Framingham Heart Study, HF patients had a 5-year survival rate of 25% in men and 38% in women, making heart failure a more lethal condition than some cancers. Mortality increases with age, is 50% higher in blacks than in whites, and one third higher in men than women. (Ho, et al., 1993) Study of the natural history of heart failure has been limited by the high percentage of patients that die suddenly from presumed lethal arrhythmia (35–50%). However, clinical observation of end-stage heart failure patients shows that a high percentage of deaths are complicated by renal failure or respiratory failure which may be secondary to long-standing heart failure or a co-morbidity.

Etiology of Symptoms

Symptoms experienced by persons with HF are from the body's compensatory mechanisms for the failing heart. The three primary compensatory mechanisms include: increased sympathetic activity, neuroendocrine activation and ventricular remodeling. In heart failure, a reduction in cardiac output results in tissue hypoperfusion and direct activation of the sympathetic nervous system. This leads to a stimulation of contractility and heart rate and vasoconstriction in areas of less metabolically active tissues such as skin, kidneys and venoconstriction. Venoconstriction increases venous return and increases preload. The decrease in renal flow results in stimulation of the renin-angiotensin-aldosterone system causing increased sodium and water retention and increased potassium excretion, which worsens vasoconstriction. This then so increases preload and afterload. The third compensation is a remodeling of the ventricle. Initially the heart dilates to preserve the amount of blood pumped out with each beat. However, dilation increases wall stress and leads to a compensatory hypertrophy. Now the ventricle is stiffer and may thicken beyond what the coronary circulation can support.

The decreasing ability of the heart muscle to put out an adequate volume of blood at an adequate pressure, coupled with prolonged systemic venous hypertension, can result in congestive hepatomegaly, ascites, varying degrees of nausea and anorexia, pleural effusion, and dependent edema. The dependent edema, sometimes called cardiac edema, will occur in the legs symmetrically in ambulatory patients, and in the sacral region of patients in bed. Pitting edema of the arms and face occurs rarely and only late in the course of heart failure.

Advanced Stage Symptoms

Most patients can be brought into a state of compensation so that symptoms of fluid-overload are kept to a minimum. The natural history of the disease is a downward spiral that is a result of remodeling of the architecture of the heart muscle. This is depicted by acute episodes but patient does not return to former function. This remodeling causes a decrease in heart function and a worsening of symptoms that results from low cardiac output and fluid overload. These symptoms require ever increasing doses of medications to return to equilibrium until the side effects of the medications finally limit the therapy that is possible. Cardinal symptoms of heart failure are dyspnea and fatigue.

Dyspnea

Patient's severity of illness is classified by determining what level of activity precipitates dyspnea. (Figure 9) Dyspnea is a result of an increased interstitial and alveolar congestion. Orthopnea, the inability to breathe while lying flat, and paroxysmal nocturnal dyspnea (PND) are slightly different manifestations of this same problem. When fluid in the lungs reaches a certain level rales may be heard at the lung bases and a wheeze may be present. However, in long standing heart failure, the lymphatic system may compensate for the high fluid load and rales may be absent despite high pressures in the pulmonary vasculature. A dry cough may be present especially when lying down.

FIGURE 9	New York Heart Association (NYHA) Functional Classification
Class I	Patients with cardiac disease, but without resulting limitation of physical activity. Ordinary physical activity does not cause undue fatigue, palpitations, dyspnea, or anginal pain.
Class II	Patients with cardiac disease resulting in slight limitation of physical activity. They are comfortable at rest. Ordinary physical activity results in fatigue, palpitation, dyspnea, or anginal pain.
Class III	Patients with marked limitation of physical activity. They are comfortable at rest. Less than ordinary activity causes fatigue, palpitation, dyspnea, or anginal pain.
Class IV	Patients with cardiac disease resulting in inability to carry on any physical activity without discomfort. Symptoms of heart failure or of the anginal syndrome may be present even at rest. If any physical activity is undertaken, discomfort is increased.

Stuart, et al., 1996.

Fatigue

Fatigue is thought to be a result of a decreased cardiac output that causes both tissue hypoxia in the exercising muscle and a sluggish vascular response to exercise. Initially, vasodilators, ACE inhibitors or Hydralazine and Isordil, can improve cardiac output and thus the patient's functional capacity. Rest and pacing activity is a lifestyle change that becomes essential. Some patients benefit from timing activity to take advantage of the period when their medication is peaking. There does come a point in the end stages of the disease where fatigue is profound and the patient will require complete assistance with all ADL's. Just prior to the point when a patient is bed-bound is the ideal time to consider a positive inotropic medication to enhance cardiac output. This is considered a palliative measure or a bridge to heart transplantation as patients have a 25% higher risk of sudden death while on these medications because of their proarrhythmic side effect. Drugs like Dopamine, Milrinone, and Dobutamine require intravenous access and continuous infusion or a short-term hospital stay for intermittent infusion. Careful assessment of the patient's family support and cognitive ability to accommodate such a therapy will determine if these drugs are appropriate options. There is no evidence that these medications prolong life but they can ameliorate low output symptoms.

Prognosis Criteria

The U.S. Department of Health and Human Services' Agency for Health Care Policy and Research (AHCPR), as well as many researchers, use the New York Heart Association (NYHA) Functional Classification in their guidelines and/or research criteria. (See Figure 9)

In the AHCPR guidelines for patients with left ventricular dysfunction, the probability of mortality using the NYHA is as follows:

    Class II   5–10%/yr
    Class III   10–20%/yr
    Class IV   20–50%/yr

Within each class, the presence of more severe or progressive symptoms, or accompanying angina would push these estimates to the higher end of the range; conversely, milder symptoms, clinical stability, and absence of angina would shift the estimate to the lower end.

According to the *Medical Guidelines for Determining Prognosis in Selected Non-Cancer Diseases* published by the National Hospice Organization (Stuart, et al., 1996); the likelihood of early mortality is increased in patients with:

- NYHA Class IV symptoms or severe heart failure symptoms at rest.
- Ejection fraction of 20% or less is helpful supplemental objective evidence, but should not be required, if not already available.
- Persistent heart failure symptoms despite maximal medical management with vasodilators and diuretics.
- A history of ventricular or symptomatic supraventricular arrhythmia resistant to antiarrhythmic therapy, cardiac arrest or unexplained syncope.
- Embolic CVA of cardiac origin.
- Concomitant HIV disease.

Heart failure patients can survive for long periods with severe symptoms, which makes determination of the optimum timing of hospice or palliative care most difficult.

Symptom Management

Interventions are focused on reducing the demand on the myocardium, since its lack of efficiency is the cause of the distressful symptoms the patient will experience. This is accomplished by reduction of the cardiac workload, enhancement of myocardial contractility, and control of excessive fluid retention. Approaches to these three components are outlined in Figure 10. Specific symptom management ideas for edema, nausea, anorexia, dyspnea and fatigue are discussed in Table 1.

In certain situations, long term technological aids that have been utilized during the course of the illness may need to be evaluated. For instance, implanted epidural pumps, implantable cardioverter defibrillators, pacemakers, etc. may create additional problems in the final hours. Decisions must be made on how and when deactivation should occur. Funeral directors should be informed to prevent problems during cremation.

FIGURE 10 | Interventions for Heart Failure

Reduction of the Cardiac Workload

Non-Prescriptive	Prescriptive
■ Reduction in physical activity. ■ Periods of rest in bed or in a chair. ■ Small frequent meals better than three large meals. ■ Weight reduction program in obese patients. ■ Psychosocial and/or medication interventions to reduce stress and anxiety.	■ Anticoagulants, leg exercises, and elastic stockings if patient on bed rest and is at risk for thrombophlebitis. ■ Mild sedation with barbiturates or tranquilizers if needed to calm the patient or permit sleep.

Enhancement of Myocardial Contractility

Non-Prescriptive	Prescriptive
■ Obtain written orders indicating both high and low parameters for holding medication; teach patient and/or family how to check rate or blood pressure before medicating. ■ Observe for signs of hypokalemia: muscle weakness, hypotension, and respiratory distress. ■ Observe for signs of digitalis toxicity: changes in heart rate, nausea & vomiting, excessive salivation, abdominal pain, confusion, and visual disturbances. ■ Observe for signs of dehydration, nausea, anorexia, headache, orthostatic hypotension, or dizziness and lightheadedness.	■ Digoxin and digitoxin are the standard cardiac glycosides used to increase the force and velocity of myocardial contraction. Patient needs to be monitored for hypokalemia, and drug interactions; some interactions will decrease the effectiveness of the glycoside, and others will increase the action—resulting in digitalis toxicity. ■ Sympathomimetic amines: epinephrine, isoproterenol and dopamine are also used for improving contractility; but would not likely be used outside acute care settings. ■ Positive inotropes such as dobutamine and milrinone can be used in the home setting but must be initiated in an acute setting.

Control of Excessive Fluid Retention

Non-Prescriptive	Prescriptive
■ Low sodium intake (2Gms/day) to decrease total body sodium stores. This can usually be achieved by not adding salt when cooking or serving and restricting high sodium foods (canned products, processed cheese and meats, boxed mixes, milk, bread, and fresh spinach, celery, and beets). ■ Restricting fluid intake may help, but is not as important as limiting sodium intake. ■ Caloric restriction in obese patients (to reduce the workload of the heart). ■ Administer diuretics in the morning to prevent sleep disruption. ■ Anticipate amount of assistance patient may need for frequent voiding. ■ Caution patient to rise slowly and pause between position changes as diuretics and ACE inhibitors may cause postural hypotension.	■ Diuretics are used to increase the urinary excretion of sodium and water. Thiazides, loop diuretics, and spironolactone are commonly used, sometimes in combinations with each other. The caution is to not overtreat; resulting hypovolemia may reduce cardiac output, interfere with renal function, and produce profound weakness and lethargy. Depending on prognosis and disease trajectory, may want to monitor electrolytes for hypokalemia or hyperkalemia and worsened renal insufficiency.

Compiled from Smith & Campine, 1984; Rich, 1997.

Renal Disease

By Debra Heidrich

Overview

Kidney diseases can be grouped into two main categories: acute renal failure or chronic renal failure. In acute renal failure, the kidneys abruptly stop working, but may eventually recover to normal function. In chronic renal failure (CRF), there is a progressive loss of kidney function, which is irreversible. The patient is considered to be in end-stage renal disease (ESRD) when the number of functioning nephrons decreases below 20 to 30 percent of normal. (Guyton & Hall, 2000) At this point, the glomerular filtration rate is likely below 10 ml/min. and dialysis or renal transplant are the remedial treatments to relieve symptoms and delay complications. (McDougal, 1996)

There are many potential causes of chronic renal failure (see Figure 11). Renal failure from these diseases occurs because of disorders of the renal blood vessels, glomeruli, tubules, renal interstitium, or lower urinary tract. The end result, no matter what the underlying cause, is a decrease in the number of functioning nephrons. Although glomerulonephritis was believed to be the most common cause of CRF, diabetes mellitus and hypertension are now recognized as the leading causes of end-stage renal failure (Guyton & Hall, 2000).

The exact incidence of renal failure is unknown, but approximately 90,000 people in the United States receive Medicare benefits for renal dialysis, with 8,000 new cases entering into the program each year. (Luckmann, 1997) Persons with ESRD on dialysis have a prognosis of 25 years or more.

FIGURE 11	Common Causes of Chronic Renal Failure

Diabetes mellitus
Hypertensive nephrosclerosis
Glomerulonephritis
—Polyarteritis nodosa
—Lupus erythematosus

Infections
—Pyelonephritis
—Tuberculosis

Nephrotoxins (analgesics, chemotherapy, antibiotics, heavy metals)
Congenital disorders
—Polycystic disease
—Congenital absence of kidney tissue

Urinary tract obstructions

Compiled from Guyton & Hall, 2000.

Pathophysiology

The kidneys filter 180 liters of fluid per day and serve multiple important physiologic and hormonal functions, including regulation of water, electrolyte and acid-base homeostasis, excretion of metabolic waste products and foreign chemicals, regulation of arterial pressure, secretion of hormones, and gluconeogenesis. (Guyton & Hall, 2000; Shapiro & Schrier, 1992; Luckmann, 1997; Woolfson & Mansell, 1994) With renal failure, the kidneys are not able to maintain this internal homeostasis, leading to multiple complications.

As renal function decreases, the remaining nephrons and their glomeruli increase in size in order to compensate. Thus, there may not be clinical signs of renal dysfunction until only about 25–30% of nephrons are functioning. Sodium excretion is generally maintained until late in the disease. At this time, the excretion of sodium becomes fixed and the kidneys are no longer able to vary excretion according to the patient's needs. While the urine output is still relatively normal, this may result in hyponatremia. When the glomerular filtration rate falls below 20 ml/min, the kidney is unable to compensate for varying water loads resulting in both water and sodium retention. The kidneys maintain the ability to excrete potassium until the glomerular filtration rate falls below 10 ml/min. At this time hyperkalemia may become evident, although it is usually not significant until the urine output is less than 500 ml/24 hours. (McDougal, 1996)

Acid-base balance may be maintained until the glomerular filtration rate falls below 20 ml/min. At that point the distal tubule is unable to maintain excretion of ammonia and other acidic end-products of metabolism. In addition, bicarbonate wasting occurs in response to fluid overload, lowering the body's capacity to buffer the retained acids. The combination of these two factors can lead to a significant metabolic acidosis.

The breakdown products of protein metabolism include urea, uric acid and creatinine. As these chemicals are excreted by the kidneys, they accumulate in proportion to the number of nephrons that have been destroyed. Therefore, the blood urea nitrogen (BUN) and creatinine clearance are relatively good indicators of renal function, although less so in the elderly. The protein-restricted "renal diet" is aimed at reducing the symptoms of uremia by decreasing the amount of protein breakdown products in the body. The dietary restriction of protein also slows the progression of renal failure. (McDougal, 1996)

Serum phosphate also rises as kidney function decreases. This causes a fall in serum calcium and a release of parathyroid hormone. The parathyroid hormone acts on the tubules to increase phosphate excretion, returning the serum phosphate to normal. But, in the process, the parathyroid hormone has caused bone reabsorption, resulting in bone destruction and depositing of calcium in soft tissues. (McDougal, 1996)

Advanced Stage Symptoms

All organ systems of the body are affected by renal failure. Many of the signs and symptoms are summarized in Table 6. Laboratory criteria for limited prognosis in ESRD patients are: (1) a creatinine clearance less than 10cc/min (less than 15 cc/min for diabetics) AND (2) a serum creatine greater than 8.0 mg/dl (greater than 6.0 mg/dl for diabetics). (Stuart, et al., 1996)

Since dialysis can prolong survival for years, it is presumed that a patient seeking hospice or specialized palliative care would not be opting for dialysis or transplant. Those persons who fit the criteria for dialysis and are refusing initiation or continuation of dialysis are generally appropriate for hospice. In addition to the laboratory confirmation of elevated serum creatine and decreased creatinine clearance (as noted above), a nephrology consult may be helpful since individual patient variables can influence longevity. The following clinical signs are the criteria for beginning dialysis, and thus, define appropriateness for hospice care (Stuart, et al., 1996):

- Clinical manifestations of uremia
  —Confusion, obtundation
  —Intractable nausea and vomiting
  —Generalized pruritis
  —Restlessness
- Oliguria: Urine output less than 400cc/24hrs
- Intractable hyperkalemia unresponsive to medical management (potassium > 7.0)
- Uremic pericarditis
- Hepatorenal syndrome
- Intractable fluid overload

The key to optimal hospice/palliative care of persons with ESRD is assessing for actual or potential uncomfortable symptoms and instituting appropriate interventions. Likely symptoms will include: peripheral neuropathy and paresthesias, nausea and vomiting, weakness, painful gout, confusion/restlessness, and edema. Interventions for these symptoms are outlined on Table 3. It should be remembered that any patient with neuropathic pain would also experience allodynia (pain to a stimulus that does usually provoke pain, such as a light touch or clothing).

Figure 12: Pathophysiology, Clinical Manifestations and Complications of Chronic Renal Failure

Pathophysiology	Clinical Manifestation	Complications
Water and salt retention	Edema; fluid overload	Hypertension (increases risk of cardiovascular and cerebrovascular disease) Dyspnea Pulmonary edema Pneumonia
Metabolic acidosis due to inability to excrete acidic products	Confusion, apathy, stupor Shortened memory/attention span Kussmaul breathing	Seizures Coma
Increase in urea, uric acid, and creatinine due to inability to excrete metabolic end-products of protein	Nausea & vomiting Anorexia Uremic breath Hyperparathyroidism Gout: swollen, painful joints Muscle wasting, weakness	Pericarditis
Metabolic disorders —including aluminum intoxication	Metallic taste Peripheral neuropathy/paresthesias Shortened memory/attention span Disturbed sleep	Agitation Seizures Psychotic behavior
Abnormal calcium and phosphorus metabolism —partially due to hyperparathyroidism	Altered bone growth and demineralization —bone pain & fracture —swollen, painful joints —soft tissue calcium deposits (brain, eyes, joints, heart, skin) —renal osteodystrophy	Bone fractures
Hyperkalemia	Myocardial dysfunction —tented T-waves, widened QRS complexes, conduction abnormalities Muscular weakness	Congestive heart failure Ventricular standstill
Crystallization of calcium salts	Decreased skin oil and sweat —itching, excoriation —brittle nails and hair	Dermatitis
Altered insulin production	Carbohydrate intolerance	Hypo/hyperglycemia
Impaired coagulation, capillary fragility	—contusion, bruises —bleeding gums —bleeding diathesis —GI bleeding —pallor	Anemia
Impaired erythropoietin production	Anemia and pallor	Poor oxygenation
Abnormal urinary tract (in some patients)	Kidney infection Bladder infection Kidney stones	Bacteremia
Inability to metabolize nutrients	Poor nutritional status Impaired wound healing	Malnutrition

Compiled from Guyton & Hall, 2000; Luckman, 1997.

TABLE 3 — Symptom Management of Renal Disease

Symptom	Non-Prescriptive	Prescriptive
Neuropathy, paresthesia, or allodynia	- Relaxation. - Distraction. - Application of heat or cold; carefully avoiding extremes. - Massage. - Avoid stimulation of allodynia, such as light touches.	- TENS (Transcutaneous electrical nerve stimulation). - Methadone is the opioid of choice for neuropathy, since it blocks n-methyl-D-aspartase receptors. Most other opioids have little benefit in neuropathic pain. - Certain anticonvulsants at appropriate doses and tricyclic antidepressants, SNRIs (Venlafaxine Nefazodone) are specific for neuropathic pain. - Capsaicin (Zostrix) cream topically should not be used long term, since it may induce toxicity.
Nausea & vomiting	- Relaxation. - Positioning. - Small frequent meals. - Decrease dietary protein.	- Antiemetic should be selected based on etiology; haloperidol may be drug of choice for uremia.
Weakness	- Goal-setting with patient so energy is conserved for most important tasks. - Utilization of family and aids to decrease energy output; home devices such as bedside commode may be appropriate. - Utilization of input from occupational or physical therapists as appropriate.	- Steroids or stimulants may increase energy in some patients for brief periods, not recommended for long-term use. - Sorbitol or IV glucose may help if weakness is related to elevated potassium. Kayexalate should rarely be used in the terminally ill due to side effects and drug interactions. - Biphosphonates (i.e. alendronate, clodronate, etidronate, ibandronate, pamidronate, risedronate, tiludronate, zoledronate) plus fluids may help if weakness is due to elevated calcium. - Avoid thiazide diuretics; furosemide may be useful if patient cannot tolerate fluid load. - Blood transfusions may be indicated for severe symptomatic anemia, depending on the patient's goals and disease trajectory. - Role of erythropoietin requires further evaluation in anemia and the palliative care setting.
Painful gout	- Warm applications locally. - Increase oral intake as appropriate to help excrete urates.	- Topical capsaicin (Zostrix); should not be used long term since it may induce toxicity. - Colchicine, NSAIDs to decrease plasma urate. - NSAIDs as analgesic if not putting kidneys at too great a risk (creatinine less than 1.5). - Trial of steroids if allergic to NSAIDs.
Confusion/restlessness	- Frequent reorientation. - Maintain quiet relaxing environment. - Minimize external stimuli. - Insure uninterrupted rest periods. - Speak directly to patient; especially to explain procedures or treatment.	- Haloperidol (Haldol). - Ativan if haloperidol ineffective. - Biphosphonates (i.e. alendronate, clodronate, etidronate, ibandronate, pamidronate, risedronate, tiludronate, zoledronate), fluids and lasix if elevated calcium is the cause.
Edema	- Fluid restriction as appropriate. - Low sodium diet as appropriate. - Positions of comfort and position changes.	- Diuretics as appropriate. - Low-dose opioid if edema is causing dyspnea.

Compiled from: Kaye 1997; Smith, 2000; Kemp, 1999; Sheehan & Forman, 1996; Woodruff, 1999; Doyle, et al., 1998; Ferrell & Coyle, 2001.

Liver Disease

By Sue Meyer, Jayne Galley-Reilley, Sheila Duffy and Debra Whitaker

Overview

The liver is the largest organ in the body and performs more than 400 functions. (Reishtein, 1993) At rest it accepts a blood supply of approximately 1300cc every minute. Between meals, more than three-quarters of this supply comes from the intestines via the portal vein.

Liver Anatomy

The liver has two main lobes; these are further divided into thousands of lobules, which are literally drenched with blood. The portal vein brings blood from the small intestine, which is low in oxygen but rich with newly absorbed nutrients. At the microanatomical level the basic functioning units are the hepatocytes. They handle nutrients arriving from the intestines, converting glucose to glycogen, manufacturing cholesterol from fats and rearranging amino acid sequences from absorbed proteins to arrive at usable forms. Hepatocytes also convert toxic substances into harmless waste products. Blood leaving the liver via the hepatic vein carries the processed nutrients to be distributed to all the tissues. The liver has a second blood supply which brings oxygenated blood to the liver tissue via the hepatic artery. This highly ordered structure of the liver is critical to its function and any disorder of its architecture can lead to disturbances.

The liver's activities affect every other organ and system in the body. Many conditions can cause hepatic dysfunction, hepatitis B and C and cirrhosis being just a few. Once liver function decreases beyond a certain level, no matter the cause, the untoward effect is the same. (Reishtein, 1993)

Liver Functions

STORAGE AND DISTRIBUTION. Amino acids derived from digestion are stored and eventually reconstructed into a variety of essential body proteins. Carbohydrates as glycogen, iron as ferritin, copper, vitamins and blood volume are stored in the liver. (Martin, 1992; Reishtein, 1993) Fat stores are regulated and the liver controls the production and excretion of cholesterol.

PRODUCTION AND SECRETION. The liver produces albumin, which functions in the maintenance of colloid osmotic pressure, and clotting proteins such as fibrinogen and prothrombin. About a liter of bile is produced in a day. It is concentrated and stored in the gallbladder to be released into the small intestine to aid in fat digestion.

CONVERSION. With a drop in blood glucose level, the liver converts stored glycogen to glucose. If glycogen reserves become depleted, fats and proteins are converted into glucose as well. Excess ingested protein is broken down into ammonia, converted into urea and excreted by the kidneys.

DETOXIFICATION. Many drugs are metabolized into active/inactive forms. Some hormones are broken down preventing their toxic buildup. The liver's Kupffer cells digest bacteria, viruses and other potentially damaging substances that arrive via the portal circulation from the intestinal tract.

Pathophysiology

Hepatitis B

Hepatitis B is caused by the hepatitis B virus (HBV). The disease is more prevalent and infectious than AIDS and is responsible for 3000–4000 deaths annually. (American Liver Foundation, 2000) The virus lives in the blood and body fluids and can remain dormant in the body for years after the initial incident of infection. Because of this, there can be a lifelong liver infection leading to cirrhosis, liver cancer, liver failure and death. Transmission is by direct contact with blood or body fluids, such as transfusions, use of contaminated needles/syringes, sexual contact or perinatal. Thirty to forty percent are acquired by unknown mechanisms. (Sherlock & Dooley, 1997c) After contact, some of those infected may fight off the disease, but approximately 10% will become carriers of the virus and another 10% will progress to chronic liver disease.

With initial infection the most common symptoms are flu-like, headache, cough, nausea, occasional diarrhea and pronounced fatigue and weight loss. In some instances, there are no symptoms at all. Within a few days jaundice develops and urine becomes dark. With the onset of jaundice symptoms may improve. Jaundice may last for a few weeks or continue many months. Lymph nodes in the neck are enlarged, joints ache, the liver and often the spleen are enlarged. (Schiff, et. al., 1999)

The diagnosis of chronic HBV is made by blood tests indicating the presence of active virus, elevated liver enzymes and decreased levels of serum albumin. (Schiff, et. al., 1999) Hepatitis B progresses to end stage liver disease (ESLD) when the diagnosis of hepatic cirrhosis is made. Hepatocellular carcinoma is a common sequella of chronic HBV. (Cooper, et al., 1997)

Hepatitis C

The major cause of transfusion related non-A; non-B hepatitis was identified in 1989 as an RNA virus, which was named hepatitis C virus (HCV). (Tong, et. al., 1995) Hepatitis C has reached epidemic proportions in the United States with approximately four million Americans infected. Hepatitis C accounts for 30% of all liver transplants in the United States each year. (Sherlock & Dooley, 1997c) In the United States intravenous drug abuse has been responsible for 60% of transmissions in the past six years with 20% of the new cases attributed to sexual transmission. (Women's Health Advocate, 1998) The rate of HCV transmission from mother to child is rare, it can be transmitted through blood contact from shared needles, as well as hygiene items such as razors, tooth brushes or scissors. Studies show that individuals living in a non-sexual living arrangement for a long period of time have an increased risk for becoming infected with the virus. (Schiff, et al., 1999) Four percent of reported cases in the United States have occurred in health care workers who have contracted the virus in the workplace.

Most patients with HCV have asymptomatic elevations in liver enzymes (AST and ALT) and no physical signs of the disease. Initial symptoms may be mild malaise or flu-like symptoms that do not impact upon the individual's activities of daily living. Other symptoms may include dull right upper quadrant pain, anorexia, weight loss, myalgia, arthralgia and fatigue. Jaundice occurs in less than 30% of HCV patients. (Sherlock & Dooley, 1997c) Chronic HCV is an indolent disease, slowly infecting a patient over many years. Transaminase fluctuations during this time are most likely due to flare-ups of HCV viremia. Most patients, however, feel only fatigue during this phase. Chronic HCV can be associated with various other disorders, such as systemic vasculitis, purpura, neuropathy, thyroiditis, or Raynaud's phenomenon. (Tong, et al., 1995)

Twenty percent of HCV positive patients develop cirrhosis. Unlike other forms of cirrhosis caused by other disease processes where bilirubin levels are elevated and indicate the level of disease progression, in HCV transmission levels tend to be a better indicator. Liver transplantation can be a viable alternative for the HCV cirrhosis patient who has no other concomitant disease process. However for many patients who do not have the option of transplantation, the disease can represent a rapid downward spiral following a diagnosis of cirrhosis from HCV.

Cirrhosis

Cirrhosis is defined as a diffuse process of hepatocellular necrosis, followed by fibrosis and nodule formation. Early fibrosis is reversible but cirrhosis with nodules is not. Distortion, twisting and constriction of central sections of lobules cause impedance of portal blood flow and that results in hepatocellular failure and portal hypertension. Approximately three fourths of the liver can be destroyed without symptoms of impairment. (Alspach & Williams, 1985; Sherlock & Dooley, 1997d) Chronic alcohol ingestion, chronic hepatitis B and C, and unknown causes may cause cirrhosis. The terminal stages of the various types may be identical.

Advanced Stage Symptoms

The clinical course of the various types of liver disease is remarkably similar. It starts with acute inflammation of the entire liver leading to hepatic cell necrosis and bile duct damage of varying degrees. (Alspach & Williams, 1985) For lack of a better definition chronic hepatitis is defined as "continuing disease without improvement for at least six months." (Desmet, et al., 1994) Cirrhosis is the final and irreversible stage of chronic hepatitis, and combines some or all of the features described below. (Sherlock & Dooley, 1997a)

General Failure of Health

The hallmark and most common symptom of chronic hepatitis is malaise or fatigue. (Desmet, et al., 1994) This is often described as extreme physically limiting tiredness. (Wainwright, 1997) Weight loss can also be dramatic. Wasting may be related to difficulty in synthesizing tissue proteins. (Sherlock & Dooley, 1997a)

Jaundice

As the liver fails and secretes less bile, bilirubin—an ingredient of bile—builds up in the blood. Jaundice becomes apparent clinically when the bilirubin rises to 3mg/dl, giving a yellow color to skin, sclera and darkening the urine. (Wallach, J.B., 2000) The stools become lighter in color from lack of bile presence. (Martin, 1992; Reishtein, 1993) When jaundice is present, it represents active hepatocellular disease and a bad prognosis; its intensity paralleling the extent of liver damage. Hemolysis of erythrocytes adds to the jaundice. (Sherlock & Dooley, 1997a) Pruritus accompanies jaundice.

Hyperdynamic Circulation and Cyanosis

This is present in all forms of liver failure but especially with decompensated cirrhosis. It is evidenced by flushed extremities, bounding pulses and capillary pulsations. Decreased plasma proteins cause a decrease in osmotic pressure that leads to generalized edema and the formation of ascites. Pooling of blood in the spleen and opening of normally closed arteriovenous anastomoses add to the size of the circulatory tree. (Reishtein, 1993) To supply the increased circulation, cardiac output increases, as evidenced by tachycardia and frequently a systolic ejection murmur. Systemic vascular resistance is low, thus the effective arterial blood volume falls as a consequence of the enlargement of the arterial vascular compartment. Hypotension follows, contributing to the downward spiral of liver failure by further decreasing hepatic and cerebral blood flow. The renin-angiotensin system becomes activated thus sodium and water is retained furthering the accumulation of ascites. (Sherlock & Dooley, 1997a)

Hypoxemia

Hypoxemia is seen in up to one third of people with cirrhosis who have no underlying heart or lung disease. (Reishtein, 1993) There is a decrease in the saturation of the hemoglobin molecule related to an increase in concentration of 2,3-diphosphoglycerate within the red blood cell and reduction of diffusing capacity due to dilatation of small pulmonary blood vessels. This results in less oxygen being picked up in the lung while more oxygen is given up to the tissues. A high diaphragm secondary to massive ascites or hepatomegaly and pleural effusions may further reduce pulmonary function. (Alspach & Williams, 1985; Reishtein, 1993; Sherlock & Dooley, 1997a)

Fever and Septicemia

Normally, the Kupffer cells of the liver filter the blood preventing intestinal bacteria from entering the systemic circulation. In cirrhosis, bacteria can reach the general circulation by passing through this faulty hepatic filter or through porto-systemic collaterals. (Reishtein, 1993; Sherlock & Dooley, 1997a) Adding to this, leukocyte function is impaired and fluid build up in edema and ascites set the stage for septicemia. Spontaneous bacterial peritonitis (SBP) is an infection of ascites fluid occurring without an obvious source. Translocation of bacteria from any source: gut, urinary tract or lung can cause bacteremia. Without the normal clearance activity of the Kuffper cells in the liver and less bacterial destruction by blood neutrophils, a transient bacteremia now can become prolonged and seed the ascites leading to SBP. (Bass, 1998) Aspiration is common in people with decreased mental function, leading to pneumonia. Urinary tract infections are particularly common as well. (Sherlock & Dooley, 1997a)

Hepatic Encephalopathy

Encephalopathy is observed in advanced liver disease and can be considered an early stage of hepatic coma. Ammonia and other substances toxic to brain cells are present in the vascular circulation because liver cirrhosis impairs the metabolizing/detoxifying functions, and because blood is forced to flow through collaterals, bypassing the liver altogether. Ammonia is the most widely investigated of these toxic substances; ninety per cent of patients with hepatic encephalopathy have elevated ammonia levels. (Alspach & Williams, 1985; Sherlock & Dooley, 1997b)

Clinical features include drowsiness, confusion, irritability, and a characteristic flapping tremor (asterixis). The onset is usually insidious with gradual changes in consciousness, personality, intellect and speech. There are, however, factors which may precipitate a more rapid onset, such as potent diuretics, large volume paracentesis, high protein intake, GI bleed, anesthesia, acute alcoholism, opiates, benzodiazepines, barbiturates, infection, severe constipation and shunting procedures. (Reishtein, 1993; Sherlock & Dooley, 1997b)

Ascites

As liver tissue becomes fibrous, lymph can no longer drain effectively. This excess fluid leaks into the peritoneal cavity and accumulates as ascites. Lowered plasma oncotic pressure, resulting from failure of the liver to synthesize albumin, contributes to the fluid buildup. (Alspach & Williams, 1985) Intravascular fluid loss triggers the renal tubules to retain sodium and water via the secretion of aldosterone. Hepatic failure may also compress the liver's blood vessels obstructing flow and causing a resistance to flow through the liver. This portal hypertension causes an increase in hydrostatic pressure within the liver leading to hyperfiltration and extravasation of fluid, further contributing to the formation of ascites. (Bass, 1998)

Changes in Nitrogen Metabolism

Liver failure disables the function of protein catabolism and subsequent conversion of the byproduct, ammonia, to urea. This results in deranged amino acid balance, a drop in serum albumin levels, and a negative nitrogen balance. The consequence of a state of negative nitrogen balance is a lack of adequate nitrogen for protein synthesis. (Reishtein, 1993) Protein is absorbed and retained but is not used for serum protein manufacture. (Sherlock & Dooley, 1997a) Plasma prothrombin and other proteins concerned in blood clotting may be deficient. Coagulopathy may be so profound in terminal liver failure that exsanguination may be caused by simple procedures.

Skin Changes

Vascular spiders appear in the vascular territory of the superior vena cava, rarely below the nipple line. These consist of a central arteriole with radiating small vessels resembling a spider's legs. Arterial spiders may disappear with improving hepatic function and conversely the appearance of new lesions suggests progression. If ruptured, spiders bleed profusely. (Alspach & Williams, 1985; Sherlock & Dooley, 1997a)

Palmar erythema is not as frequently seen in cirrhosis as are vascular spiders but both may be present. The hands are warm and palms bright red in color. Many normal healthy people have familial palmar flushing. Both spiders and palmar erythema have been attributed to estrogen excess or an abnormal ratio between estrogens and androgens. (Sherlock & Dooley, 1997a)

Bleeding and Varices

As the liver fails, its ability to synthesize vitamin K and various clotting factors falters and an elevated prothrombin time and thrombocytopenia results in a high risk for bleeding. (Alspach & Williams, 1985; Martin, 1992) Resistance to blood flow is high in fibrotic distorted livers. Blood shunted through collateral vessels that connect the portal veins to those supplying other organs causes portal hypertension. The shunting of blood through the small veins at the esophagogastric junction produces distention and hypertrophy. (Alspach & Williams, 1985) These enlarged and tortuous vessels, called varices, are subject to erosion by stomach acid and mechanical trauma. A sudden increase in abdominal pressure, i.e. from coughing, straining or vomiting may result in bleeding. Bleeding in this area combined with a loss of clotting control is disastrous and often fatal.

Symptom Management

The person dying from liver failure is dying from multisystem failure, since the actions of the liver affect every other organ and system; the circulatory system, the respiratory system, and the renal system, to name a few. For many of these patients, the cause of death is often a relatively sudden and unpredictable event such as bronchopneumonia, sepsis, cardiac arrhythmia or gastrointestinal hemorrhage. (Fox, et al., 1999) For others, death may occur quietly and peacefully as they lapse into a fatal coma.

In earlier stages when there is hope for remissions and extended periods of wellness, efforts are made to control or slow the disease process. For example, alcoholic cirrhosis can have dramatic improvement if the patient chooses complete abstinence. Many patients with hepatitis C respond well to treatment with alpha interferon. Liver transplantation can be a viable option for the HCV cirrhosis patient who has no other concomitant disease process. Corrective treatment for acid-base imbalance, electrolyte imbalance, and nutritional supplementation may be administered to slow the increasing spiral of pathophysiology.

In some cases, symptomatic treatment of associated symptoms such as pruritus is the only therapeutic goal, whereas in others a more aggressive approach, such as placement of a biliary stent through a gross stricture, may markedly improve the quality and perhaps even the duration of life. (Bain & Minuk, 1998)

In more advanced stages, the pain and dyspnea of ascites may be relieved by paracentesis. Attempts may be made to control hemorrhage of esophageal varices by insertion of ballooning tubes, or by administration of vasopressin. Whether or not these and other aggressive treatments are performed should depend on the patient's goals, and whether any particular treatment offers any benefit that offsets the burden. Sometimes that decision cannot be made until the recommended treatment is given a trial to determine the degree of benefit and burden of side effects.

The cause of hepatic failure is important to prognosis and potential for treatment response. For example, the patient with jaundice due to extensive hepatic infiltration with malignant cells may have only weeks to live, while in other patients, jaundice and resulting pruritis may be eased by simple measures such as stopping a hepatoxic medication or a low protein diet. The severity of symptoms and the disease trajectory also impacts the potential of certain treatment decisions. The *Medical Guidelines for Determining Prognosis in Selected Non-Cancer Diseases*, published by the National Hospice and Palliative Care Organization (Stuart, et al., 1996), suggest parameters that indicate a limited prognosis in hepatic disease:

- Patient is not a candidate for liver transplantation
- Impaired liver function shown by both of the following:
  —Prothrombin time prolonged >5 sec. over control
  —Serum albumin <2.5 Gm/dl
- Clinical indicators of end-stage liver disease (any one of the following):
  —Ascites refractory to sodium restriction and diuretics: spironolactone 75–150 mg/day
  PLUS furosemide > 40 mg/day
  —Spontaneous bacterial peritonitis
  —Hepatorenal syndrome (cirrhosis and ascites, elevated creatinine and BUN, oliguria <400 ml/day, and urine sodium concentration < 10 mEq/L)
  —Hepatic encephalopathy refractory to protein restriction and lactulose or neomycin therapy
  —Recurrent variceal bleeding despite injection sclerotherapy, oral beta blockers, transjugular intrahepatic portosystemic shunt (TIPS), or patient refusal of further therapy
- Factors shown to worsen prognosis if present:
  —Progressive malnutrition
  —Muscle wasting with reduced strength and endurance
  —Continued active alcoholism
  —Hepatocellular carcinoma
  —HbsAg positivity

Regardless of stages of disease, comfort measures for distressing symptoms should be administered. These are outlined in Table 4.

TABLE 4 Symptom Management of Liver Disease

Symptom	Non-Prescriptive	Prescriptive
Pruritis	■ Cool air (reduces sweating and lessens itch). ■ Avoid hot baths and drinks that cause vasodilation (alcohol, hot caffeine drinks). ■ Moisturizing lotions and bath oils. ■ Starch or oatmeal baths. ■ Avoid soaps or applications containing alcohol (causes drying). ■ Loose fitting cotton clothing. ■ Short nails and cotton gloves if patient scratching. ■ Ice pack to local area of severe episodic itching. ■ Distraction activities (boredom makes itch more noticeable).	■ Topical therapy: preparations containing menthol, camphor, phenol, zinc oxide, calamine, doxepin, or corticosteroids. ■ Cholestyremine (Questran), 4 Gm qid to remove bile acids. ■ Antihistamines: hydroxyzine (Vistaril), diphenhydramine (Benadryl), or chlorpheniramine (Chlor-Trimeton). The bedtime dose should be a sedating dose. (Waller & Caroline, 1996)
Agitation, hallucinations and psychosis from encephalopathy	■ Reassuring presence of a familiar person. ■ Brief and simple explanations about surroundings, people present, and care procedures. ■ Calm atmosphere with minimal stimuli. ■ Assess a confused patient for urinary and bowel problems.	■ Reduce ammonia levels (Woodruff, 1999): —Restricted dietary protein. —Oral lactulose, 30 ml q8h until 2–3 soft stools/day, or —Neomycin, 1 Gm daily. ■ Treat agitation: (Consult psychiatry) —Diazepam (Valium) or other benzodiazepam. ■ Treat hallucinations and psychosis: (Consult psychiatry) —Haloperidol (Haldol).
Dyspnea and pain from ascites	■ Position for comfort and maximum diaphragm excursion; usually with upper torso elevated. ■ Plan care and activities to minimize exertional dyspnea. ■ Move air in room by fan or open window.	■ Diruretics: spironolactone, 100 mg q am (increasing stepwise to 200 mg bid if needed) *and* furosemide, 40 mg q am (increasing stepwise to 240 mg q am if needed). (Waller & Caroline, 1996) ■ Low dose morphine for dyspnea: morphine sulfate, 5 mg SC or 10–15 mg PO q3h PRN. ■ Effective pain management. (Refer to a). ■ Paracentesis (Refer to b). ≤ 5 L/day (Doyle, Hanks & MacDonald, 1998); possibly followed by instillation of bleomycin or other sclerosing agent. ■ Peritoneovenous shunt (Refer to b) (LeVeen or Denver) depending on patient goals and prognosis, and nature of ascites; works poorly if fluid is bloody, viscous or loculated. (Woodruff, 1999)

(continued)

Symptom	Non-Prescriptive	Prescriptive
Nausea, vomiting, and early satiety	■ Offer small frequent meals. ■ Allow patient to self-regulate intake. ■ Cold foods may be more appealing. ■ Assess for relationship of nausea to specific drugs or activities. ■ Eliminate strong or repulsive odors. Provide restful environment; ascertain and deal with anxieties.	■ Discontinue offending drugs if possible. ■ Oral lactulose, 30 ml q8h. ■ If gastric irritation component, give H_2 histamine receptor antagonist (cimetidine, ranitidine). ■ Antiemetics: prochlorperazine (Compazine), haloperidol (Haldol), etc. (Refer to c).
Fatigue or discomfort from infections	■ Decrease demands on patient, encourage periods of rest as needed. ■ May use cool cloths to forehead, armpits or groin if temperature increases.	■ Antibiotic therapy as indicated depending on prognosis, potential for improving patient comfort, gaining functional status, or extending meaningful time. (Refer to d).

Compiled from: Kaye, 1997; Smith, 2000; Kemp, 1999; Sheehan & Forman, 1996; Woodruff, 1999; Doyle, et al., 1998; Ferrell & Coyle, 2001.

a) Since patients with liver disease will have impaired metabolism, administration of hypnotics, analgesics, and sedatives must be carefully considered. For example, long-acting short-chain barbiturates (i.e., phenobarbitol) are preferred over short-acting long-chain drugs, because the former are not dependent on the liver for metabolism/detoxification. Meperidine (Demerol) is not usually recommended for end-stage pain. Morphine is not contraindicated in renal or hepatic dysfunction, but needs close observation in titrating the dose; a lower dose and longer dose interval may be necessary to get desired effect without opioid toxicity. (Doyle, Hanks & MacDonald, 1998)

b) Invasive procedures in end stage liver disease have high potential for infection and bleeding.

c) Haloperidol is a useful drug as it is a strong antiemetic causing low sedation, less anticholinergic, and minimal cardiac and CNS side effects compared to phenothiazines.

d) Fever is a common symptom in many end-stage diseases and is not always distressful to the patient. Palliative care should be aimed at comfort goals for the individual patient, not correction of a problem, e.g., an elevated temperature.

Neurological Diseases

By Noreen Leahy

Amyotrophic Lateral Sclerosis

Overview

Amyotrophic Lateral Sclerosis (ALS), also known as Lou Gehrig's Disease, is a progressive degenerative disease affecting motor neurons in the spinal cord, brain stem and motor cortex of the brain. Amyotrophic refers to the muscle atrophy, that results from degeneration of the motor neurons, while lateral sclerosis refers to the gliotic scarring, or sclerosis, of the voluntary motor pathways of the corticospinal and corticobulbar tracts. (Barker, 1994) The disease is characterized by muscular weakness and atrophy while sensory disturbances and sphincter control are usually spared. (Adams, et al., 1997)

The annual incidence in the United States is about 1.4 per 100,000 people, with men affected slightly more than women, and the onset occurring during or after the sixth decade. (Adams, et al., 1999) While the etiology is unknown, theories abound and factors include: viral, bacterial, metabolic, neurotoxins, heavy metals, minerals, hormones, and an impaired immune system. (Barker, 1994) Approximately 5% of those afflicted inherit the disorder as an autosomal dominant trait. (Adams, et al., 1997) The course of the disease is such that the average life span from the onset of symptoms to death is about 3 years. (Barker, 1994)

Pathophysiology

The degenerative processes affect the anterior horn cells of the spinal cord, the motor nuclei of the brain stem, the corticospinal tract, and the motor neurons of the cerebral cortex. The upper motor neuron involvement produces decreased muscle strength, spasticity, and hyperreflexia, while lower motor neuron involvement is demonstrated by flaccidity, atrophy, and paralysis. Electrical and chemical impulses from upper motor neurons to lower motor neurons are disrupted as the motor neurons degenerate. It is known that there is excessive glutamate (one of the main CNS excitatory neurotransmitters) activity in the brain and spinal cord of these patients, but the underlying reason is unknown. (Carter, et al., 1999)

Early signs may vary but include weakness, wasting and cramping of hand muscles resulting in loss of facility in performing fine motor activities, and fasciculations (an incoordinate contraction of skeletal muscle in which groups of muscle fibers innervated by the same neuron contract together) of the forearm, upper arm and shoulder. Involvement of the face, jaw, tongue, pharyngeal, and laryngeal musculature early in the disease course generally heralds a very progressive disease course. (Adams, et al., 1997) As the disease progresses, muscle strength and bulk decline. A common presentation is one in which there is atrophy and weakness of the upper extremities, slight spasticity of legs and arms, and hyperreflexia.

Dysarthria (impairment of articulation) progresses to the point where speech may be unintelligible at first, then absent. Slurring of speech is attributed to weakness and/or spasticity of the muscles involved in articulation. To help decrease the frustration and anxiety over the inability to communicate, it is best to establish alternative means of communication early.

Drooling and difficulty swallowing occur as a direct result of impaired motility of the tongue, pharynx, and esophagus, and from facial muscle weakness. Thin fluids and chunky foods can cause choking and aspiration. Adapting the diet to incorporate high caloric foods that are easy to chew and swallow is necessary. The expertise of a speech therapist is very helpful in teaching alternative swallowing techniques. (Borasio & Voltz, 1997) Decisions concerning artificial nutrition and hydration are discussed in Table 1 in the section on "General Signs and Symptoms."

Sensation remains intact, there is no involvement of the autonomic nervous system, and cognitive function is unaffected. Because mentation remains intact throughout the progression of ALS, some degree of depression is common. Clinically significant depression can occur at any stage of the disease, and antidepressant drug therapy may be indicated. Antidepressant drugs can be useful in this population, not only for depression per se, but also for the sedative and anticholinergic beneficial side effects. (Enck, 1994) It is important to differentiate between normal reactive depression, pseudobulbar affect (spontaneous uncontrollable episodes of inappropriate laughter or crying), and simple sadness/frustration. The former two benefit from antidepressant therapy, the latter may benefit more from psychosocial interventions (especially if the sedative and anticholinergic effects of the drugs are not desirable). Management of depression is discussed in Table 1 in the section on General Signs and Symptoms.

Advanced Disease

Weakness is the initial major functional limitation, with endurance fluctuating on a daily basis. As the disease progresses, the complaint of "heaviness" is supplanted by paresis and eventually paralysis. Coarse fasciculations of the extremities eventually cease as the muscle becomes totally denervated. Discomfort from muscle cramping is not uncommon and is due to the degeneration of the motor axons.

Individuals in the terminal stages of ALS typically appear cachectic with severe muscle wasting. Confusion, restlessness, and lethargy may be seen as hypercapnea becomes more pronounced. Advanced stage of the disease is marked by involvement of the brainstem motor nuclei, producing atrophy and weakness of the neck, tongue, pharyngeal and laryngeal musculature. The end-stage of ALS is demonstrated by the involvement of the respiratory musculature, causing death by aspiration or respiratory failure.

Because there is great variability in disease progression, multiple clinical parameters and clinical judgment are required to judge the progression of ALS. However, a prognosis of months (not years) can generally be expected when patients fit one of the following categories (Stuart, et al., 1996):

1) *Both* rapid progression of ALS (progressing from independence to needing major assistance in ambulation and ADLs in past 12 months) *and* critically impaired ventilatory capacity (vital capacity less than 30% of predicted, with significant dyspnea at rest with supplemental O_2).

2) *Both* rapid progression of ALS *and* critical nutritional impairment (continued weight loss plus dehydration and/or hypovolemia), with a decision not to receive artificial feeding.
3) *Both* rapid progression of ALS *and* life-threatening complications (recurrent aspiration pneumonia, fever despite antibiotics, infected stage 3–4 decubitus ulcers, etc.).

Symptom Management

Since there are no curative treatments for ALS, palliative care begins at the time of diagnosis. Only one drug, riluzole (inhibits glutaminergic neurotransmission) is FDA approved for treatment of ALS. It does not cure the disease, but may add three months to longevity. (Carter, et al., 1999) Information needs to be conveyed to the patient and family at appropriate intervals so that they are aware of potential course of symptoms and potential outcomes of treatment choices. Because the progression of the disease produces a heavy psychological burden on both the patient and the caregiver, there needs to be a plan for psychosocial support. Before the physical condition declines to requiring total care, discussions need to occur to determine what supports will be needed if the patient is to remain at home.

Physical therapy is an invaluable resource in providing exercises and recommendations to prevent muscle contractures and joint stiffness. High toilet seats, tub lifts, and wheelchairs are all likely to be necessary to facilitate daily activities as the course of the disease progresses. Use of an electric hospital bed will allow for both better positioning and easier transfers to and from the bed. Transfer techniques should be taught to the individual and the caretaker in order to prevent injury to either person. Increased immobility and decreased nutritional status make the patient more susceptible to soft tissue breakdown; this is discussed in Table 1.

The expertise of an occupational therapist is paramount in identifying adaptive devices to assist with upper extremity activities such as eating, bathing, and dressing, as well as modifications that can support the individual in the home. Additionally, energy sparing and pacing techniques can be taught to the individual to maximize energy expenditures. Other symptoms are discussed in Table 5.

Multiple Sclerosis

Overview

Multiple Sclerosis (MS) is a chronic, progressive, and degenerative disease that affects the conduction pathways of the central nervous system. Characteristically it presents with a multitude of symptoms and its course is marked by periods of exacerbation and remission, with the severity and duration of the exacerbation increasing as the disease progresses. While the etiology is unknown, it is postulated that genetic susceptibility, environmental exposures, and an autoimmune response may all combine in some manner to cause the disease. (Goroll, et al., 1997)

It is more common in the northern latitudes and the highest rate of incidence is between ages 20 and 40, with an incidence 2–3 times higher in women. (Adams, et al., 1997) There is a well established familial tendency, with approximately 15 percent having an affected relative. (Ebers, 1983)

Pathophysiology

MS causes demyelination of the myelin sheaths (sometimes referred to as the "white matter") that encompass the axons or long conduction pathways within the central nervous system. The affected area is infiltrated by lymphocytes, macrophages, and plasma cells that produce an inflammatory process, which in turn results in the development of a sclerotic plaque or scar. The resultant demyelination is usually focal, disrupts the electrical transmission of impulses, and most commonly affects the optic nerves, spinal cord, brainstem, cerebellum, and periventricular areas. Symptoms may resolve with the resolution of the inflammatory response, and over time, some partial remyelination of the axon may occur. (Adams, et al., 1997) These episodes of the central nervous system may remit and recur over a period of 20 to 30 or more years. Precipitating factors include various types of infection, emotional trauma, injury, and pregnancy. Eventually nerve fibers degenerate, and symptoms become permanent.

In general, the disease may follow one of three models. Younger persons tend to develop a *relapsing and remitting* course, characterized by complete or near complete remission following an attack. These individuals may go on in later years to develop a *chronic/progressive* course that is manifested by a gradual worsening and commonly, involvement of the spinal cord. A *relapsing/progressing* course marks a more severe form of the disease characterized by acute attacks with little remission. (Goroll, et al., 1997) The life expectancy is predicated upon the form of the disease an individual has, age at onset, their response to current treatment modalities, and the presence of concomitant systemic problems. Because of the scattering of sclerotic plaques throughout the nervous system, symptoms may vary widely from one individual to another.

Ocular Symptoms
- Optic neuritis or clouding of the central visual field and transient pain upon eye movement
- Nystagmus
- Diplopia with or without ocular muscle palsies

Motor Symptoms
- Complaint of weakness or heaviness in the lower extremities
- May worsen spontaneously or be due to precipitating factors such as exercise or changes in temperature
- Incoordination—fine motor activities of the hands may become almost impossible to execute; voluntary movement becomes ataxic
- Dysarthria (impairment of articulation) due to involvement of the muscles of speech
- Severe spasticity and contractures may be evident
- Severe motor weakness may give rise to respiratory complications of atelectasis, pneumonia, and failure

Sensory Symptoms
- Numbness and tingling may occur on the face or any of the involved extremities
- Proprioception and joint sensation are often diminished and accompanied by sensations of constriction as well as edema
- Pain is uncommon, though discomfort from spasticity and contractures may be present
- L'hermitte sign is a phenomenon described as an "electric-shock like" sensation down the shoulders and back produced with passive flexion of the neck

Cerebellar Symptoms
- Scanning speech (slow and measured)
- Rhythmic instability of the head and neck
- Intention tremor of the extremities
- Incoordination of voluntary movements and gait
- Charcot's triad, manifested by nystagmus, scanning speech, and intention tremor is often seen in the advanced stages of the disease

Acoustic Nerve Symptoms
- Vertigo or a slight sensation of instability may be an early presenting symptom
- Nausea, vomiting and nystagmus may accompany the vertigo as portions of the VIIIth cranial nerve are affected

Mental Status Changes
- Cognitive dysfunction: confusion, distractibility, word finding difficulty
- Emotional lability ranging from depression to euphoria

Bowel and Bladder Symptoms
- Fecal incontinence, constipation, impaction
- Neurogenic bladder may present as urgency, hesitancy, incontinence, or retention

Advanced Disease

In the last stages, the patient is bedridden, usually incontinent, may have painful flexor spasms of the lower extremities, and usually has recurrent febrile episodes from infections (bladder, lung, decubiti, etc.). Palliative care is the main focus of treatment from the time of diagnosis since there is no curative treatment for multiple sclerosis. It is difficult to judge when the prognosis makes the patient eligible for hospice consideration. This decision would have to be based on a combination of factors such as the general guidelines for determining limited prognosis found in the introduction to this monograph, clinical judgment of someone familiar with the case, and consideration of the patient's goals and values. The stress and strain of a long-term roller coaster illness with ever-increasing care needs places a tremendous burden on the caregivers/family members. Considering that this could be lasting over a period of several decades, there is a high indication for psychosocial support and ways to provide respite to caregivers.

Symptom Management

General support includes encouragement of bedrest in acute exacerbations, and planning to prevent excessive fatigue. As the disease progresses, the same assessment as for ALS should be made to determine proper assists to maintain independence and safety. As nutritional status and mobility decreases, meticulous attention should be paid to the prevention of bedsores by the use of alternating pressure mattresses, silicone gel pads, and other special products and devices to relieve pressure, and prevent abrading and poor circulation. The only specific medicinal treatment found to stimulate return to recovery from acute episodes is steroids. This is usually used for several days and then tapered. A few patients may be kept on small doses every other day for several months. The disadvantage of prolonged steroid therapy is potassium depletion, euphoria/depression, insomnia, bone mass depletion, peripheral edema, gastritis, and acne.

The symptom of emotional lability (either responding inappropriately or not being able to stop crying or laughing) can be upsetting to patient and family. It is helpful to explain to patient and family that this is a usual part of the disease. Explain that it is a physical impairment of voluntary control over emotions; it is not purposeful, nor is it a sign of any change in mental or cognitive function. It is best to remain calm, matter-of-fact, and reassuring during the episode.

Because constipation is a common problem, a preventive bowel regime/bowel training program should be instituted. Further symptom management ideas will be found in Table 1 and Table 5.

Cerebrovascular Accident (CVA)

Overview

Stroke continues to be the third leading cause of death in the United States, following heart disease and cancer. It is defined as a sudden, nonconvulsive, focal neurological deficit that develops abruptly. (Adams, et al., 1997) It develops as a result of a pathologic process that develops over time. Epidemiological studies have identified numerous risk factors for stroke, many of which are controllable. Among the most important are hypertension, heart disease, atrial fibrillation, diabetes mellitus, long-standing history of cigarette smoking, and hyperlipidemia. Familial history, the use of oral contraceptives, and presence of systemic diseases which produce a hypercoagulable state are also identified risk factors.

In the United States, there are about 500,000 individuals each year who suffer strokes, with a fatal outcome occurring in approximately 175,000 of these people. (Adams, et al., 1997) The frequency of stroke increases with age, doubling for every decade after age 55; and strokes occur more often in women and African-Americans than Caucasians. Mortality figures range from 17–34 percent during the first month after the event, and from 20–40 percent during the first year. (Gresham, et al., 1995) The aggregate lifetime cost of stroke is estimated to be $29 billion. (Taylor, Davis, Torner, et al., 1996)

Pathophysiology

Stroke can be categorized into two main classifications: ischemic and hemorrhagic. The neurological deficit produced reflects the location and extent of the ischemia or hemorrhage. The pathophysiology associated with ischemic strokes is based on the interruption of oxygen and glucose supply to the cells, leading to subsequent interruption of basic cellular processes that cause neuronal death. The major events leading to ischemic strokes are thromboses and emboli.

Ischemic Strokes

Thrombotic strokes occur as the arterial lumen becomes progressively occluded over time. Contributing causes may include atheromatous plaque formation, hypercoagulability states, and hypoperfusion. Individuals may present with the stroke in evolution, such that neurological deficit continues to increase in severity over the course of hours or days, or maximal infarction may have already occurred by the time of presentation. Transient ischemic attacks (TIAs) may herald thrombotic events in some persons, producing neurological deficits demonstrative of the affected brain tissue.

Embolic strokes occur much more rapidly as they result from occlusion of cerebral vasculature from circulating particles. Individuals with atrial fibrillation or flutter are at high risk for embolizing a blood clot to the brain. Additional sources of emboli include stenotic lesions of the carotid artery, septic debris, fat, and microparticulate matter from cardiac, orthopedic or vascular surgery.

Hemorrhagic Strokes

Hemorrhagic strokes occur with bleeding into the intracranial vault or directly into the brain parenchyma. Extravasation of blood creates a mass that compresses the adjacent brain structures, may extend into the ventricular system, and may cause shifting of midline structures and compromise of the vital brain stem centers. (Adams, et al., 1997) Edema also contributes to the picture as it increases during the first few hours, as well as hydrocephalus due to compression of the ventricles. Hypertension is a common predisposer; the integrity of the vessel is disrupted from constant high pressures, with bleeding occurring into the tissue and/or surrounding subarachnoid space. Hemorrhage into the subarachnoid space may also occur from ruptured cerebral aneurysms or arteriovenous malformations.

Strokes and Cancer

CVAs are a fairly common complication of end-stage cancer; 14.6% in one study (Obbens, 1998), usually related to tumor, tumor treatment, or coagulation disorders such as thrombocytopenia with or without disseminated intravascular coagulation (DIC). The treatment depends on the underlying cause, such as coagulopathy or cerebral metastasis; in either case, the prognosis is not good.

Advanced Stage Symptoms

With catastrophic strokes, the individual is generally comatose. Extremities are flaccid, the individual is unresponsive to noxious stimuli, or reacts with abnormal decerebrate or decorticate posturing. Pupil size may be unequal, or fixed in position and sluggish or non-reactive to light. Respirations may be deep, irregular, or intermittent. Impaired consciousness or impaired gag and swallow reflexes place the individual at risk for airway obstruction and aspiration and their sequelae.

Poor outcomes can be expected when large areas of the brain have been infarcted, or when intracerebral clots are greater than 30 ml in volume. (Adams, et al., 1997) The summary of studies related to survival of CVAs by Stuart, et al., (1996) found the following as strong predictors of early mortality:

- Coma or persistent vegetative state secondary to stroke beyond 3 days' duration.
- Patients with any 4 of the following present on day 3 of comatosed state: abnormal brainstem response, absent verbal response, absent withdrawal response to pain, serum creatinine > 1.5 mg/dl, or age > 70.
- Dysphagia severe enough to preclude oral intake, in a patient who declines or is not a candidate for artificial nutrition and hydration.

Patients who survive the acute episode tend to stabilize with supportive and rehabilitative care. The pattern from this point may be maintenance of functional level, with future morbidities and/or mortality from other etiologies; or recurrent stroke or periodic TIAs. In a chronic or subsequent phase of CVA, the following clinical factors correlate with poor survival: (Stuart, et al., 1996)

- Age > 70.
- Poor functional status: Karnofsky score < 50%.
- Post-stroke dementia, as evidenced by a FAST score of > 7 (See Figure 13).
- Poor nutritional status, whether on artificial nutrition or not:
  - Unintentional progressive weight loss of > 10% over past 6 months.
  - Serum albumin < 2.5 mg/dl (never a sole indicator).

In addition to the above, the factors known to apply to any debilitated patient with progressive clinical decline may apply, such as: aspiration pneumonia, pyelonephritis, sepsis, refractory stage 3–4 decubitus ulcers, or recurrent fevers despite antibiotics.

Management of Symptoms

As indicated in the above discussion, if patients survive the acute CVA episode, they may continue to manage well with supportive measures and die much later from declining chronic disease or from an entirely different disease entity. Treatment during the intervening period, whether that is months or years, will consist of supportive, rehabilitative and preventive measures to maintain optimal functioning and quality of life. Management of general neurological symptoms is presented in Table 5.

FIGURE 13 | Functional Assessment Staging (FAST)

(Check highest consecutive level of disability)

1. No difficulty either subjectively or objectively.
2. Complains of forgetting location of objects. Subjective work difficulties.
3. Decreased job functioning evident to co-workers. Difficulty in traveling to new locations. Decreased organizational capacity.
4. Decreased ability to perform complex tasks, e.g. planning dinner for guests, handling personal finances (such as forgetting to pay bills), difficulty marketing, etc.
5. Requires assistance in choosing proper clothing to wear for the day, season, or occasion, e.g. patient may wear the same clothing repeatedly unless supervised.
6.
    a) Improperly putting on clothes without assistance or cueing (e.g. may put street clothes on over night clothes, or put shoes on wrong feet, or have difficulty buttoning clothing) occasionally or more frequently over the past weeks.
    b) Unable to bathe properly (e.g. difficulty adjusting bath-water temperature) occasionally or more frequently over the past weeks.
    c) Inability to handle mechanics of toileting (e.g. forgets to flush the toilet, does not wipe properly or properly dispose of toilet tissue) occasionally or more frequently over the past weeks.
    d) Urinary incontinence (occasionally or more frequently over the past weeks).
    e) Fecal incontinence (occasionally or more frequently over the past weeks).
7.
    a) Ability to speak limited to approximately a half dozen intelligible different words or fewer, in the course of an average day or in the course of an intensive interview.
    b) Speech ability is limited to the use of a single intelligible word in an average day or in the course of an intensive interview (the person may repeat the word over and over).
    c) Ambulatory ability is lost (cannot walk without personal assistance).
    d) Cannot sit up without assistance (e.g. the individual will fall over if there are not lateral rests {arms} on the chair).
    e) Loss of ability to smile.
    f) Loss of ability to hold up head independently.

Reisberg, B. 1988.

TABLE 5 Management of Neurological Symptoms

Symptom	Non-Prescriptive	Prescriptive
Communication deficit/impaired articulation of speech	■ Discuss communication options if possible; personal preferences of patient will work best. ■ Ascertain best time of day for important communications; it is usually mornings. ■ Allow pauses for periods of rest. ■ Avoid raising your voice or "talking down" to patient, when their mental capacity and hearing remains the same. ■ Use communication boards with pertinent pictures or words. ■ Use computers with special controls. ■ Encourage patient to talk "telegraph" style: short phrases. Confirm each word to be sure you have understood correctly. ■ Visit patient often as there may be fear of distress without means of getting help. ■ Carry on interactions only when in front of and at face level with the patient. Their faces can be very expressive and communication can happen without speech.	■ Speech Therapist will suggest speech exercises, as well as aids to swallowing.
Spasticity, muscle weakness, tremors, atrophy	■ Work with therapist to determine best transfer techniques, passive exercises, splints and other supports to maintain positions of function, i.e., roll to support hand position or footboard to prevent footdrop. ■ Teach and encourage caregivers to carry out passive exercises. ■ Teach patient relaxation exercises; very useful when respiratory muscles are affected. (Saunders, et al., 1981)	■ Physiotherapy: exercises to prevent flexion contractures and to assist range of motion to enhance independent activities of daily living (ADLs). ■ For muscle spasm: —Diazepam (Valium), 5–10 mgm HS. —Baclofen 5–30 mgm TID pc (is less sedating than benzodiazepines; dose should be increased slowly to avoid nausea and drowsiness). (Kaye, 1989)
Drooling	■ Provide ample supply of tissues, folded towels, bibs, etc. ■ Position with head elevated and turned to side to reduce choking episodes. ■ Hand-held suction device to capture excessive saliva.	■ Anticholinergics (hyoscyamine, scopalamine, atropine) to decrease secretions; with precaution that long-term use can affect vision and/or render sputum too viscous. (Saunders, et al., 1981)
Seizures	■ Protect patient from injury during seizure (never forcefully restrain); to prevent tongue from obstructing airway, roll on side or insert oral airway. ■ Observe for ataxia or over-sedation as side effects of diazepam. ■ Hold food, liquids, or oral medications until patient is fully alert; postictal period can last for varying periods of time. ■ Provide calm atmosphere (low levels of noise, confusion, or bright lights).	■ Prevention therapy is usually phenytoin 100 mg TID or Dilantin 300 mgm QD; or use of valproic acid (Depakote) or carbamazepine (Tegretol). ■ If oral administration is a problem, phenobarbital can be given in a rectal suppository, IM or as a continuous subcutaneous (SC) infusion. ■ Focal or generalized seizures best controlled by diazepam (PR or SL) or lorazepam.

Compiled from: Kaye, 1997; Smith, 2000; Kemp, 1999; Sheehan & Forman, 1996; Woodruff, 1999; Doyle, et al., 1998; Ferrell & Coyle, 2001.

Dementia

By Sally Smith

Overview

Dementia is a syndrome that involves permanent loss of intellectual functions and memory sufficient to impair activities of daily living. Cognitive losses occur in any or all of the following domains: memory, language, visuospatial skills, complex cognition, and emotion and personality. (Bolla, et al., 2000; Klein & Kowall, 1998) Dementia is a serious health care problem in this country with an estimated 4 million Americans suffering with Alzheimer's disease or an associated progressive degenerative dementia. In one study, researchers found that over 10% of a community population over the age of 65 had probable Alzheimer's disease. (Evans, et al., 1989) The prevalence rate for those 65 to 74 years of age was 3%, those 75 to 84, 18.7% and for those over 85, 47.2% were affected.

Pathophysiology

There are four major types of progressive degenerative dementia based on the neuropathological changes that occur in the central nervous system: Dementia of the Alzheimer Type, Vascular Dementia, Diffuse Lewy Body Dementia and Pick's Disease. (Bolla, et al., 2000; Klein & Kowall, 1998) Dementia of the Alzheimer Type (DAT) is the most common illness, accounting for approximately fifty percent of all dementias. Neurofibrillary tangles and senile plaques destroy the cerebral cortex, producing atrophy. Vascular Dementia (VaD), sometimes known as multi-infarct dementia, is caused by vascular insufficiency to the brain causing multiple small and/or large infarcts. Five to 10% of all progressive dementias are of vascular origin. Diffuse Lewy Body Disease (DLBD) is now believed to be the second most common degenerative dementia causing at least 15% of all dementia. Lewy bodies are intracellular inclusions (minute foreign particles) that occur in the brain of patients with Parkinson's disease causing movement disorders. It is now recognized that Lewy bodies also occur in the cerebral cortex causing progressive dementia. Picks' Disease (PD) and/or fronto-temporal dementia account for another 15% of all degenerative dementia. The progressive atrophy of the frontal and temporal lobes of the brain, causing personality changes and socially inappropriate behaviors characterize PD. Other causes account for the remaining 10% of dementia. (Bolla, et al., 2000; Klein & Kowall, 1998)

The basic process accounting for the symptoms of dementia in all of the above illnesses is the permanent loss of neurons. At this time, there is no effective treatment to cure or arrest the progression of any of the progressive degenerative dementias. Medications, which prevent the breakdown of acetylcholine, may help slow the progression of dementia for a period of time. Unfortunately, these medications are of little help in late stage dementia.

Advanced Stage Symptoms

The course of DAT can range from 3 to 20 years but the average length of a dementing illness is 8 to 10 years. (Small, et al., 1997) In the early and middle stages of these various dementias, the presentation and treatment vary depending on the type of the dementia. In the late and terminal stages of progressive dementia, patients are more similar. They are dependent in activities of daily living, requiring the assistance of caregivers to survive. Expressive and receptive communication is severely impaired and often limited to single words or nonsense phrases. The ability to walk is lost, followed by the ability to stand, maintain sitting posture and then head and neck control. Muscle rigidity and deconditioning may lead to contractures. The ability to recognize food, self-feed, and swallow efficiently is also progressively lost, requiring skillful feeding by caregivers to prevent aspiration and/or weight loss. Incontinence of bowel and bladder occurs and skin breakdown may result. Persons with late dementia eventually do not recognize themselves or their closest friends and family. Ultimately, the ability to make eye contact is lost. The behavioral issues, which exist in the late or terminal stages of dementia, are most often anxiety or resistiveness to care due to the patient's inability to understand his environment and his need for care.

Causes of Death

The most common cause of death of patients with advanced progressive dementia is infection. As the severity of the dementia increases, the chance of developing a life threatening infection increases. Patients with late stage dementia are particularly prone to infection for several reasons: impaired immune function, immobility, incontinence, and skin breakdown that provides an entry site for bacteria. Persons who are immobile are 3.4 times more likely to develop a urinary tract infection and 6.6 times more likely to develop a lower respiratory tract infection than one who is ambulatory. As swallowing becomes increasingly impaired with advancing dementia, food or secretions may be aspirated and pneumonia may develop. (Volicer, et al., 1998)

There is little in the literature that describes the dying process of the Alzheimer patient. The dying process has been described as a transitional course for both patient and family in which the patient "fades away." (Reimer, et al., 1991) However, research with dying patients is demonstrating common patterns. In their study of terminally ill elders, McCracken and Gerdsen (1991) concluded that the terminal phase of life begins when the dying individual starts to turn from the outside world and withdraws into the internal self, thus conserving energy. The dying process observed by McCracken and Gerdsen lasted for a mean duration of 21 days. In a retrospective study at an inpatient unit for palliative care for Alzheimer patients, there was a time span of 5 to 38 days in which the nurse's notes indicated that the patient was in a dying process. (Volicer & Hurley, 1998; Smith, 1998) This time span was measured from the first nursing documentation of one of the signs of the dying process, usually food refusal, to the time of the patient's death. Figure 14 summarizes the incidence and time frames of common symptoms.

Figure 14: Incidence and Time Frames for Common Symptoms Observed in Dying Patients with Alzheimer's Disease

Symptom	% of Patients	Days Prior to Death
Decreased Appetite	100%	5–38 days
Unable to Swallow	100%	1–4 days
Lethargy	67%	5–17 days
Cardiovascular Changes (heart rate & rhythm, blood pressure, mottling)	100%	1–15 days
Renal Changes (decreased output)	80%	1–4 days
Respiratory Changes (rate, rhythm, secretions, cough)	80%	1–19 days
Musculoskeletal Changes (weakness)	100%	4–6 days
Gastrointestinal Changes (decreased bowel sounds, constipation, nausea & vomiting, incontinence)	20%	5–6 days
Mental Status Changes	67%	1–2 days

Compiled from Volicer & Hurley, 1998.

Prognosis

Since the progression of dementia to death is highly unpredictable, and because dementia itself does not cause death, prognostication is a challenge. A group of physicians who are specialists in end-of-life care reviewed existing literature to summarize some guidelines that may be helpful in identifying a patient with limited prognosis. (Stuart, et al., 1996) They suggest that if *all* of the following criteria are present, it is likely that the patient meets the prognosis of six months or less as currently required for the Medicare Hospice Benefit at or beyond stage seven on FAST Scale (see Figure 13):

- Unable to ambulate without assistance.
- Unable to dress without assistance.
- Unable to bathe properly.
- Urinary and fecal incontinence.
- Unable to speak or communicate meaningfully.
- Comorbid conditions such as repeated infections.
- Difficulty swallowing or refusal to eat.
- Unintentional progressive weight loss of >10% over prior six months and serum albumin < 2.5 Gm/dl (if on tube feeding or if tube feeding is refused).

Further, their review reveals that the presence of medical comorbid conditions (aspiration pneumonia, upper urinary tract infection, septicemia, multiple advanced decubiti, or fever recurrent after antibiotics) within the past year, further decrease survival time. Patients with difficulty swallowing or refusal to eat, coupled with refusal of artificially provided nutrition, obviously have a short prognosis. Even with these guidelines, it is not uncommon for a patient with advanced dementia and several comorbid conditions to plateau and stabilize for a year or two prior to death.

Management of Symptoms

Palliative/hospice care strives to provide the patient with maximum comfort by increasing nursing, recreational, and other pleasurable interventions while minimizing aggressive medical interventions that may cause discomfort. The degree to which medical interventions are minimized is based on the decisions reached at a family meeting in which care options *and* their potential outcomes are described to the health care proxy or family members. (Volicer, et al., 1986) In a 1993 survey, Luchins and Hanrahan (1993) found that the majority of gerontology professionals and family members of dementia patients would choose the least aggressive level of care for end-stage dementia patients. This shift from aggressive medical interventions to palliative care does not mean that the patient will receive less care. In fact, each patient receives intensive attention to comfort during the inevitable dying process, with high touch care replacing high-tech care within the context of an interdisciplinary team approach.

The dementia patient who is terminally ill presents quite differently from a non-demented patient with a terminal illness. Patients with advanced dementia are unaware of their condition and are unable to participate in care decisions. The burden of decision making is placed on the next of kin or the health care proxy. In addition, the person with dementia may behave in ways that make caregiving difficult. Anxiety, agitation, hallucinations, delusions, paranoia and aggression may all be present as care is "imposed" on the patient who cannot understand or agree with the need for care.

More importantly, patients with advanced dementia are not able to report symptoms to caregivers, hampering the diagnosis and prompt treatment of symptoms. Restlessness, unpleasant vocalizations, unwillingness to move, food refusal, aggression, changes in the vital signs and altered facial expression are some of the possible clues to discomfort in a patient who cannot verbalize it. (Hurley, et al., 1992) Staff or family caregivers may require training in special approaches and communication skills to care for demented individuals who may respond to caregiving efforts by resisting or appearing uncaring or uncooperative.

Grief intervention by the palliative care team is especially important for the families of dying dementia patients. (Rheaume & Brown, 1998) The family of the dying demented patient has special needs due to the disruptive effects of progressive dementia on family relationships. Because of the nature of dementia, the family is deprived of the opportunity to share and receive support from the demented patient as the end of life approaches. Family members are confronted with the fact that unresolved issues, which remain in the relationship from years ago, will never be resolved. Years of stressful caregiving can impair successful grieving for the spouse of a dying dementia patient.

Management of symptoms mentioned on Figure 14 is covered in Table 1. Basic principles for any patient with dementia are providing for safety without undue restraint, and minimizing external stimuli (noise, music, TV, bright lights, or any changes in the environment).

Head Trauma

By Jean Fahey

Overview

Each year in the US 150,000 deaths are attributed to trauma. It is estimated that half are due to fatal head injury. (Brain Trauma Foundation, 1998) Head injury causes more deaths and disability than any other neurological cause in persons under the age of fifty. Mortality from severe injury approaches 50% and is only slightly reduced by treatment. Head injury has no age bias. Slips and falls, child abuse, motorized vehicle accidents, bicycle accidents and violent assaults make up the majority of cases. Males are involved in twice as many head injuries and are three times as likely to die than females. The effects are not confined to the victims, but affect families and society in general. These often-preventable accidents usually involve a previously healthy individual. Severity of the insult depends on the type of injury, degree of damage, concurrent health status, and treatment options available.

Pathophysiology

The brain houses an estimated 100 billion neurons and can carry impulses up to 400 feet a second. Even minute injuries to the brain can have devastating consequences. The brain is a soft pliable mass covered by three meningeal layers and a water wrap of cerebral spinal fluid. The delicate structures are protected in a bony vault. All neuronal tracts exit and enter the brain through the foramen magnum, at the skull base.

The vascular system has a rich blood supply within these meningeal layers and deep within the brain to nourish the incredible explosion of activity that is experienced as we interact with our environment every day. The shape and thickness of the cranial bones are designed to accommodate the internal structures. The frontal bone is equipped with sinuses that act as bumpers from direct frontal assaults. The occipital bone protecting the back of the head is thick and takes a great deal of force to fracture. The floor of the brain consists of three fossas, or recesses, to accommodate the intricate structures that lie deep within the cortex and brain stem. In the pediatric population the brain is more pliable and can accommodate pressure changes because of the open fontanels and the ability of the bones to overlap each other.

Initial Trauma

Trauma to the head causes the cortex to hit against the hard skull under the point of impact. The force causes the brain to bounce inside the skull and hit the opposite pole causing damage in that area also (coup-contrecoup injury). As the cortex moves, the very delicate communication pathways in the stationary brain stem get twisted, torn, and sheared. Neurons and blood vessels are stretched and rupture. As the brain shifts from the external force the structures in the skull base are scraped along the irregular ridges and grooves in the different fossas causing more stretching, tearing and rupturing of neurons, blood vessels and meningeal

Head Trauma

layers. Frontal fractures allow a host of infectious agents from the sinuses to be released into the central nervous system.

Secondary Brain Damage

It is now clear that only part of the damage to the brain during head trauma occurs at the moment of impact. Numerous secondary insults compound the initial damage in the ensuing hours and days. The cerebral vault encases three substances, brain tissue (80%), cerebral spinal fluid (10%), and blood (10%). If one component increases, it is at the expense of the other two. Hemorrhages and widespread cerebral edema act as expanding lesions and increase intracranial pressure. The brain compensates for these increases by pushing on the less resistant compartments within the skull (see Figure 15). The opposing hemisphere is compressed and midline structures shift. The cortex pushes down resulting in brain stem compression. As the pressure increases in the lower brain stem, structures are forced through the foramen magnum, medullary function is compromised and the body's vital centers arrest.

FIGURE 15

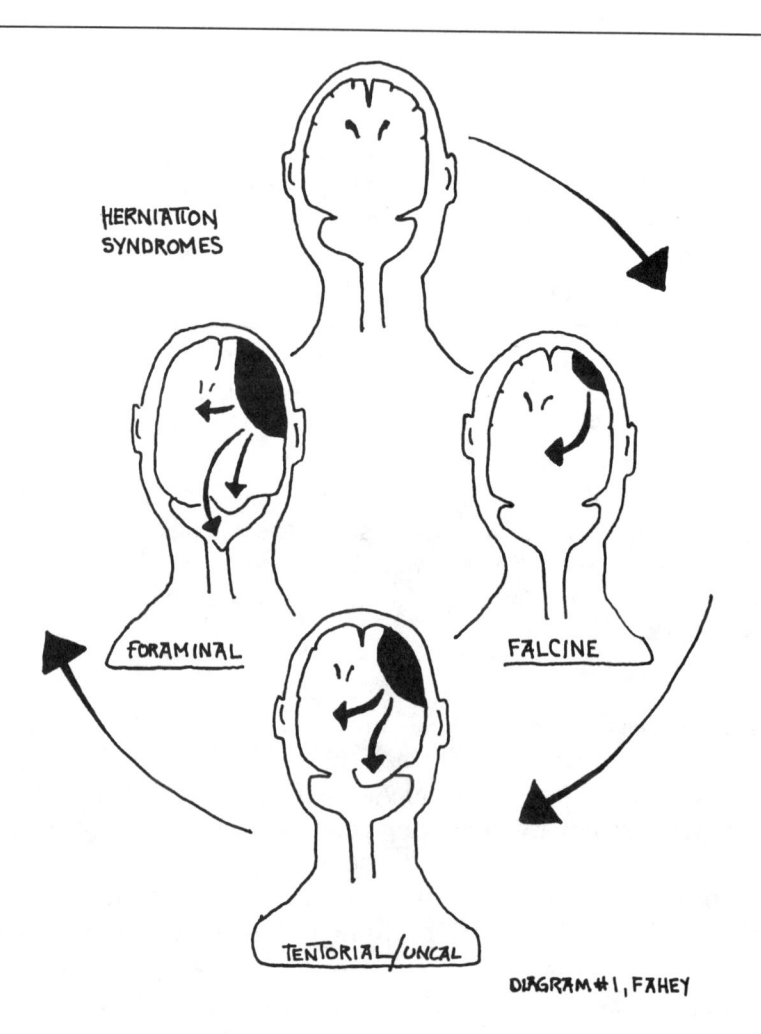

HERNIATION SYNDROMES

FORAMINAL

FALCINE

TENTORIAL/UNCAL

DIAGRAM #1, FAHEY

Advanced Stage Symptoms

Signs of increasing intracranial pressure generally progress in a rostral to caudal (head to tail) fashion. Early signs of changes in consciousness are restlessness, irritability, confusion, disorientation, difficulty following commands, difficulty verbalizing, and distractibility with normal alertness. Often the early signs go unseen, as pressures rise rapidly with acute lesions. As midline structures shift, the level of consciousness will begin to change with drowsiness and apathy. As the brain stem becomes compressed there is rapid neurologic decline starting with an ipsilateral dilated pupil. Patients become obtunded (decreased alertness or hypersomnia) or stuporous (unresponsive, but roused briefly by repeated and vigorous stimuli). Pupils progress to become bilaterally fixed and dilated. The patient will be unarousable and unresponsive. The ability of the eyes to track and focus is lost and pupils stay midline. Corneal and blink reflexes cannot be elicited and the cough and gag reflexes are lost. Responses to pain are nonpurposeful, with decorticate posturing progressing to decerebrate posturing (see Figure 16), and eventual areflexia. Respiratory decline rapidly ensues with Cheyne-Stokes respirations (deep, then shallow breaths, with periods of apnea), central breathing (deep breathing with periods of apnea) and finally ataxic breathing (gasping) until final arrest.

Management of Patients with Head Injury

The first priority of treatment for the head injured patient is complete and rapid physiologic resuscitation. (Brain Trauma Foundation, 1998) Patients are intubated at the scene or immediately upon arrival to the emergency room. Aggressive measures to reduce intracranial pressure are instituted.

Palliative care with severe head injury will depend on the phase of the injury. Consultation with palliative care specialists can guide treatment decisions and family support. General concerns common to all are pain control, symptom management, information sharing, psychosocial and spiritual support, and coordination of care. (Billings, 1998)

Ethical Considerations

Withdrawal of care from brain trauma patients differs from general medical patients in some ways. Medical patients usually face issues of physiologic futility and impending death from an incurable disease. Conversely, families of patients with brain injury must weigh the pros and cons of sustaining the body in light of little or no potential for brain recovery. Multiple life sustaining interventions frequently apply to medical patients (e.g. hemodialysis, vasopressors, and antibiotics), and treatments are often withdrawn in a stepwise fashion, with withdrawal of ventilation being the final step. By contrast, the crucial intervention for head trauma patients is almost always mechanical ventilation. Lastly, head trauma patients are most often comatose, and less often hemodynamically unstable, which may affect duration of survival and the need for medication to maintain comfort after extubation. (Mayer & Kossoff, 1999)

Palliative care in the acute care setting may consist of discontinuing vasopressors, hydration, nutrition, terminal weaning and/or extubation, which can be professionally traumatic. It is important to remind colleagues that a consensus has formed among ethicists that there is no moral distinction between not beginning mechanical ventilation and discontinuing mechanical ventilation already in use. (President's Commission For the Study of Ethical Problems, 1983) This consensus is reflected in the statements of several professional organizations including the American Medical Association, American College of Physicians, Society of Critical Care Medicine, and the American Thoracic Association.

Family Meeting

It is important for staff professionals to sit down with family members to ascertain if they have adequate information about the physiologic consequences of the injury and potential, however limited, for recovery. It may take more than one meeting, or at least a space of time, for the reality of the situation to be acknowledged. There must be great sensitivity to the shock reaction when a sudden traumatic event has occurred. Empathy and patience should affect every interaction. In some situations, as in persistent vegetative state with no chance for recovery, the decision may be made by the family to remove life support. In the case of brain death by accepted or current neurologic criteria, the family must make the decision whether or not to grant permission of tissue or organ donation, in which case the ventilator would remain until such procedures are completed.

Preparation for Removing Ventilator

Once the decision is made to withdraw ventilation, the choice between terminal weaning and extubation is made. Some practitioners prefer extubation because it is more direct. Opponents claim that failure to protect the airway risks causing respiratory distress. Reasons for preferring terminal weaning includes patient comfort and family perception. Alternatively, opponents reason it can protract the dying process. (Faber-Langedoen, 1994; Gilligan & Raffin, 1996) Dialing down the ventilator settings, either immediately or over a period of a few minutes, combines the respective advantages of extubation and terminal weaning while avoiding their pitfalls. (Gilligan & Raffin, 1996) The order and timing should be patient specific.

The process of terminal weaning includes ethical, legal and practical considerations. Two reasons terminal weaning might be recommended would include the patient's informed consent or the indication of medical futility. Clear, comprehensive and honest communications with family, guardian or surrogates must precede these recommendations. Medical futility is determined by whether the intervention is unable to prevent dependence on intensive care or if the physician has concluded the intervention had no value in the past 100 cases.

Terminal weaning is a process, not the single act of "pulling the plug" and therefore the patient/family considerations are paramount. Throughout the process, the healthcare provider is obligated to address any physical or psycho-emotional needs of the patient and family.

Reassurances begin with early discussions determining the patient's desired treatment goals accompanied by a sense of moral stability. Treatment choice disagreements may exist between patient/family and the healthcare team. Some reasons identified by Hafemeister and Hannaford (1996) are:

- the healthcare staff has not elicited the beliefs and feelings of the patient or the patient's family and friends.

- The patient, family members, or friends are unwilling or unable to listen or respond to information provided by the healthcare staff.
- Pre-existing intra-family disagreements have left family members deeply divided.
- Participants in the decision-making process have spent insufficient time discussing the decision.
- Family members and friends are frustrated by the healthcare system in general or by the course of the patient's condition, especially following a long illness.
- Treatment by a multitude of providers or frequent changes in the assigned providers, caused by fragmentation or specialization in the patient's care, has resulted in confusion, conflicting messages, and lost confidence.
- Different people simply reach different conclusions at different times based on their own dispositions, backgrounds, and experiences.
- Cultural, ethnic, and religious differences among participants in the decision-making process have become a source of conflict.

Discomforts during the terminal weaning process may include dyspnea, fear of abandonment, and anxiety. Management of these discomforts includes medications, positioning, reassurances and support of family as well as other healthcare team members. Discussion of non abandonment and the provision of explanations about what to expect, offering preference choices whether to be present/absent and offering a comfortable environment are all valuable at this time.

Determining brain death and subsequent discontinuance of life support presents an intense challenge for clinicians. A recently healthy individual lies in an intensive care bed. When one looks beyond the presence of the endotracheal tube and various lines used for care the individual appears to be simply sleeping. The electrocardiogram and blood pressure recordings are rhythmically displayed across the monitors. The chest rises and falls with ventilation. Skin color and warmth is normal, and pulses can be felt. This is the cruel reality of death in disguise. (Fahey, 1996) The determination of death by neurologic criteria, in the face of so much apparent life, creates a stressful situation for the family and the entire health care team. The focus is now not on patient comfort, as the patient has already died, but emphasis is on education and support of the family.

Organ Donation

Early consultation to the regional organ procurement agency can facilitate family support and education regarding brain death by neurologic damage and its irreversibility. As present technology is capable of sustaining cardiac function after death, these donors are sometimes referred to as "heart-beating donors." The option of organ/tissue donation may seem unpalatable under these circumstances, but the subsequent positive aspects of helping those who need transplants can give solace in the setting of a sudden, senseless death. (Bartucci & Bishop, 1987; Batten & Prottas, 1987; Fahey, 1996) However, staff should be supportive of family whether or not they decide to donate organs. When organ donation is not an option, discontinuing ventilatory support results in immediate respiratory arrest.

There is the option of tissue donation after the heart has stopped beating. In some select medical centers organs have been obtained after the heart has stopped beating as well. Within a very brief period of time after arrest a specialized team cannulates the femoral vein and infuses preservatives as the patient is taken immediately to the operating room for organ retrieval.

Nurses play an important role in preparing an environment that supports and comforts the patient and the family. This includes preparation of the physical area, preparation of the family, preparation of the patient, and preparation of follow-up. These interventions are outlined in Figure 17. Staff debriefing should also be carried out within 24 hours.

FIGURE 16

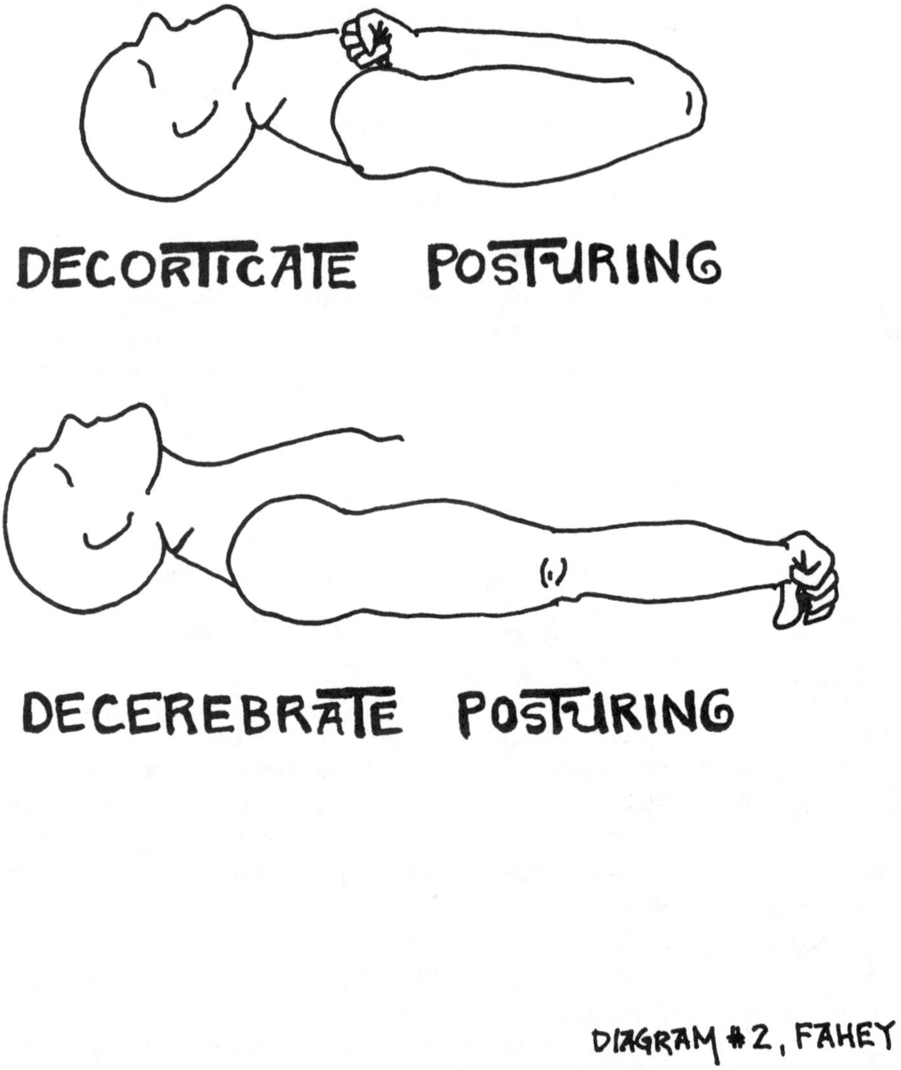

DECORTICATE POSTURING

DECEREBRATE POSTURING

DIAGRAM #2, FAHEY

FIGURE 17 | Management of Ventilator Removal

Preparation of the physical area—Non-Prescriptive

- Remove unnecessary equipment.
- Remove nasogastric tubes and any monitoring lines connected to patient.
- Turn off all monitors or alarm machines, except for the IV pump, which is necessary for delivery of analgesics and sedation.
- Remove restraints.
- Have tissues and chairs available.
- Place bed in low position so families can reach the patient's hand and head with ease.
- Advise other personnel in the immediate area so they can be sensitive to the situation.

Preparation of the family—Non-Prescriptive

- Ascertain if family members have received adequate information about condition, options, or any other concerns.
- Visitation should be as often and as long as the family desires.
- Visitations by minor children should be decided by the family; children may need special attention to their questions or fears; feelings of exclusion are often worse than feelings of sadness.
- If families desire to stay in the room when ventilator is discontinued, they should be told ahead of time what to expect (including a plan for management of patients who continue to breathe after ventilator is removed).
- Family may or may not want spiritual support or other support person present at this time.

Preparation of the patient

Non-Prescriptive	Prescriptive
- Due to unresponsive state of the patient, focus on reflexive signs such as grimacing, tachypnea, inspiratory retractions, hypertension, noisy snorting respirations, or tachycardia to assess distress. - Immediately prior to extubation, hold a clean towel in one hand as the tube is withdrawn with the other; the tube can be covered from view and any secretions wiped from the patient's mouth. - At least one staff person should remain with patient and family as long as they need to be there. - Positioning on side or gentle pharyngeal suctioning may relieve the rattling sound with respirations (when the patient is unable to clear secretions from the trachea).	- Maintain IV line for administering analgesics and sedation. - Premedicate patient if there is likelihood of the patient exhibiting distress. - Sedatives should be ready at the bedside in the event of distressing tachypnea after extubation, or during weaning. - Morphine is the drug of choice to relieve dyspnea or tachypnea (respiratory rate should be lowered to 15–20/minute). - Midazolam (Versed) or diazepam (Valium) are drugs of choice to treat multifocal myoclonus or seizures. - Anticholinergics (hyoscine, atropine, and scopolamine) should be ordered if patient has noisy respirations; it will not dry up existing secretions, but will prevent further buildup.

Preparation for follow-up—Non-Prescriptive

- Offer presence: listen when pain, anger or frustration is expressed (not necessary to "have the answer").
- May be necessary to assist family in verbalizing their questions.
- Ask if you can be of help in any way.
- Allow privacy without the family feeling abandoned.
- Assist in transfer of patient to a palliative care setting (in cases where the patient does not have neurologic brain death criteria, and continues breathing after the ventilator is removed).
- Before family leaves the room the final time, give them a paper with the MD or RN's name and phone number written out, so they can call with further questions.
- Ideally, a bereavement letter/card should be sent in the next few days.
- Offer spiritual or other psychosocial support to the family before their departure from the unit.

Fahey, 1996.

HIV/AIDS

By Kathleen Neill

Overview

The relentless spread of Acquired Immune Deficiency Syndrome (AIDS), and its causative agent, Human Immunodeficiency Virus (HIV), has caused over 13.9 million deaths pan-globally, while another 33.4 million people live with the disease. In 1998 alone, over 5.8 million people were infected with HIV, and more than 2.5 million people died of causes related to HIV. (Robbins, 1999) In the United States, there have been 420,201 cumulative deaths of all ages reported as due to AIDS, and 711,344 reported cases of AIDS. (CDC, 1999) It should be of note that these numbers probably represent under-reporting.

Changing Patterns of Incidence

As AIDS has continued to scourge the world, populations affected by the plague have begun to change. In the early days of the epidemic, HIV was primarily a disease affecting homosexual, white males. At the beginning of the 21st Century, heterosexual transmission accounts for an increasing number of AIDS cases across the United States. From 1987 to 1996 the proportion of heterosexual transmission rose from 4.8% to 17.7%. (Robbins, 1999) Intravenous drug use (IDU) or having a partner who uses IDU accounts for one half of all new infections. (Robbins, 1999)

During the early 1990s, AIDS was the leading cause of death among American men aged 25 to 44, and the 3rd leading cause of death among women of the same age group, accounting for 19.9% and 7.3%, respectively. (CDC, 1996) Among United States residents with AIDS, blacks accounted for a larger part of AIDS cases (41%) than whites (38%) for the first time in 1996. In the United States, it is estimated that between 650,000 and 900,000 people are living with HIV, and one-third of that number are unaware of their HIV disease. (Robbins, 1999)

In 1996, there was a 12% decline in AIDS incidence, but the number of persons living with AIDS, or prevalence, increased 13%. (Robbins, 1999) During the following year the Centers for Disease Control and Prevention (CDC) noted that the death rate due to AIDS had fallen for the first time. However, this decline does not signify that fewer people are becoming infected with HIV, but rather, with advances in medicopharmacologic treatment, persons infected with HIV are living longer. (CDC, 1999)

Changing Patterns of Survival

The initiation and use of highly active antiretroviral therapy, commonly referred to as HAART (see Figure 18), has enabled persons with AIDS (PWAs) to extend their lives and experience fewer episodes of opportunistic infections (OIs). Chronicity of survival thus allows both patients and health care workers to focus attention upon improving the quality of life for patients, a goal that is at the core of both palliative care and the hospice movement.

FIGURE 18	HAART (Highly Active Anti-Retroviral Therapy)

HAART is the therapy, composed of multiple anti-HIV drugs (usually 3–5), that is prescribed to limit immune damage and to fortify early immune response to HIV infection. The therapy consists of one nucleoside analog (DNA chain terminator), one protease inhibitor and either a second nucleoside analog ("nuke") or a non-nucleoside reverse transcription inhibitor (NNRTI).

Nucleoside analogs:
Zidovudine (AZT, ZDV, Retrovir), didanosine (ddI, Videx), zalcitabine (ddC, HIVID), stuvudine (d4T, Zerit), lamivudine (3TC).

Protease inhibitors (PIs):
Saquinavir (Invirase), ritonavir (Norvir), indinavir (Crixivan), nelfinavir (Viracept).

Non-Nucleoside reverse transcription inhibitors (NNRTI):
Efavirenz (Sustiva), delavirdine (Rescriptor), nevirapine (Viramune).

Compiled from Selwyn & Arnold, 1998.

Pathophysiology

HIV infection involves the complex interplay of viral replication and immune defenses. The natural history of HIV infection is divided into stages based on CD4 cell counts and clinical symptoms. After transmission, acute or primary infection can result in (but not always) the symptomatic manifestation of "acute retroviral syndrome" resembling infectious mononucleosis accompanied by high-grade HIV viremia. This is followed by seemingly spontaneous recovery in 1–3 weeks. Seroconversion generally takes place 6–12 weeks after transmission. The patient is then usually asymptomatic for an extended period, usually 10 years in an untreated patient, followed by a gradual decline in CD4 cell counts and an increasing viral load. (Bartlett, 1999)

The virus affects virtually every organ of the body, generally with multiple serious syndromes occurring simultaneously. The destruction of CD4 cells reduces the immune system making the person highly susceptible to infections. Early symptoms include opportunistic bacterial pneumonitis, vaginal candidiasis, thrush, and shingles. Pneumocystis pneumonia, toxoplasmosis encephalitis, disseminated cytomegalovirus, and mycobacterium avium complex may occur later in the disease progression.

Patients with HIV/AIDS have an increased susceptibility to cancer, the two most common being Kaposi's sarcoma and B-cell lymphomas. Patients with HIV who develop these cancers have a much higher morbidity and mortality than patients who are HIV-negative. Kaposi's sarcoma (KS) in the general population is considered a rare cancer, is usually in older men, affects the lower extremities, and usually is not the cause of death. In patients with HIV disease Kaposi's sarcoma is more common, can be systemic and widespread, responds poorly to treatments, and complications of KS can potentially be fatal. (Woodruff, 1999, pp. 379–381)

Advanced Stage Symptoms

Persons with HIV/AIDS often experience severe cachexia, extreme weakness, gastrointestinal problems, and the obvious presence of infection. Pomerantz and Harrison (1990) identified 11 common symptoms seen in end-stage HIV illness as pain, diarrhea, nausea and vomiting, dehydration, urinary incontinence, fever, respiratory problems which include chest pain, cough, and hypoxemia, skin disorders, delirium and dementia, weight loss, and depression. Patients may suffer from more than one of these symptoms at the same time, often complicating therapy.

Pain

Pain in patients with HIV/AIDS occurs from myriad factors, and is often classified as related to the disease process, related to HIV therapies, or unrelated to either HIV disease or treatment. (Hewitt, McDonald & Portnoy, 1997; Breitbart & McDonald, 1996) Disease related pain could be caused by malignancy, e.g. Kaposi's sarcoma, OIs, such as candida esophagitis, and pain due to peripheral neuropathy. Pain caused by HIV therapy includes peripheral neuropathies due to use of the medications didanosine (ddI, Videx) and ddC zalcitabine (ddC, Hivid), and procedural pain as in biopsies and radiation. Disc disease or diabetic neuropathies are examples of pain unrelated to either HIV disease or treatment.

Diarrhea

Various causes of diarrhea are diet, bacterial or viral infections of the lower gastrointestinal (GI) tract, protozoa or parasites, chronic infection, malignancies including Kaposi's sarcoma and lymphoma, and inflammatory processes such as costochondritis or cardiomyopathy. (Bresnahan & Ballou, 1999) HIV-related medications frequently causing diarrhea include antibiotics, didanosine, ddI or Videx, and the protease inhibitor nelfinavir, Viracept.

Nausea and Vomiting

Causes of nausea and vomiting include neoplasms or opportunistic infections of the GI tract; common occurrences in HIV disease. Simple food intolerance, systemic infections, pain, stress, fear, anxiety or chemotherapy side effects may precipitate nausea and/or vomiting. (Ungvarski & Schmidt, 1995) Many medications used in the treatment of HIV may induce nausea and vomiting, especially in the first weeks of beginning treatment. The protease inhibitors indinavir (Crixivan), and ritonavir (Norvir) are particularly noted for this side effect, as are the nucleoside analogues zidovodine (Retrovir) and didanosine (Videx). (Newshan & Sherman, 1999)

Dehydration

Vomiting, fever, diarrhea, and night sweats are among the causes of dehydration. Malignancies such as Kaposi's sarcoma and lymphoma may cause obstruction leading to dehydration. Candida fungal infections of the mouth and throat, aphthous ulcers, and oral Kaposi's sarcoma may make drinking fluids difficult and painful. (Bresnahan & Ballou, 1999) Ordinarily, as we have discussed in previous sections, dehydration associated with incurable illness evolving gradually over a period of weeks is not distressful to the patient. Treatment is indicated only if the patient requests it. (Kaye, 1997) In the case of HIV disease, it is somewhat different in that there are sudden and large volume losses that may recur over many months, which may call for different considerations.

Fever

Fever is not considered a serious symptom in end-stage incurable illness unless it is making the patient uncomfortable. For example, in end-stage cancer, some patients experience what is called "tumor fever." If the patient is not uncomfortable, there is no indication to initiate interventions, except to explain to the family what is occurring. However, in persons living with AIDS, fever could be one of the first signs of a change in status, an opportunistic infection, progression of the HIV disease, malignancy, autoimmune disorders, or diarrhea and dehydration. "Drug fevers" also may occur due to allergic responses to two medications frequently used in AIDS therapy, amphotericin B and trimethoprin-sulfamethoxazole. (Newshan & Arnold, 1999)

Respiratory Problems

Dyspnea and cough may be caused by bacterial, fungal, protozoan, or viral infections of the respiratory system. Lymphoma and Kaposi's sarcoma invasion of the respiratory tract may also result in dyspnea and cough. Pneumothorax, asthma and chronic bronchitis, and pulmonary embolism may precede dyspnea and cough. Simple environmental factors may precipitate cough, with or without dyspnea, while debilitation, congestive heart failure, and anemia may present in dyspnea without cough. (Newshan & Arnold, 1999; Ungvarski & Schmidt, 1995) The symptoms of dyspnea and cough are covered in Table 1 in the section on General Signs and Symptoms.

Skin Disorders

Some dermatologic diseases have a high correlation with HIV disease, such as eosinophilic folliculitis, molluscum contagiosum, or bacillary angiomatosis. Atopic dermatitis, Kaposi's sarcoma lesions and psoriasis are also manifested in persons with advanced HIV disease. Mucous membrane lesions may include aphthous ulcers, esophageal candidiasis, and Kaposi's sarcoma lesions. (Johnson, 1999)

The psychosocial ramifications of skin disorders in people with HIV/AIDS, who are already stigmatized by their HIV-positive status, cannot be minimized. Cutaneous and mucosal complications of HIV disease occur in nearly all individuals with HIV infection, may be the first presenting sign, and can be debilitating, disfiguring, and life-threatening. (Johnson, 1999) Skin conditions may improve with the use of HAART. However, side effects of the medications may cause eczematous dermatitis, possibly resulting in change of HAART regimens, and therefore decreasing the number of medications available to a patient.

Delirium and Dementia

Dementia can occur at any stage of HIV infection, and with any CD4 count, but is more common with advanced, untreated disease. AIDS Dementia Syndrome (ADS), a syndrome "which is characterized by cognitive, motor, and behavioral dysfunction" (Price & Brew, 1997, p. 334), is less common than it was in the earlier days of the epidemic due, in part, to the development of drugs which cross the blood-brain barrier. Zidovudine (AZT, Retrovir), stuvudine (d4T, Zerit), and all the non-nucleoside reverse transcriptase inhibitors: nevirapine (Viramune), delavirdine (Rescriptor), and efavirenz (Sustiva) penetrate the central nervous system. Differentiation from depression may be difficult, usually established by history of progressive cognitive deterioration, other CNS signs, and exclusion of alternative causes such as metabolic disorders, OI's, or neurosyphilis. (Bartlett, 1999)

Weight Loss

Wasting, the most insidious form of weight loss, results in a profound loss of lean body mass, and an impaired immune function with reduced resistance to infection. In turn, "Depleted lean body mass can lead to protein energy malnutrition (PEM), muscle weakness, organ failure and death." (Moscardini, et al., 1997, p. 35) AIDS wasting is generally seen in persons with end-stage disease who are not in treatment or who are failing therapy. (Gallant, 2000) Anorexia caused by many factors including side effects of medications, odynophagia/dysphagia, nausea/vomiting, lethargy and weakness, and depression contributes to weight loss and wasting. Malabsorption due to bacterial, viral, and parasitic illness also influences food intake and weight, as do diseases of the endocrine system. (Moscardini, et al., 1997) Weight loss, anorexia and cachexia are discussed in Table 1 under General Signs and Symptoms.

Depression, Anxiety, Fear, and the Lazarus Syndrome

It is estimated that "Up to 20% of HIV infected patients suffer from major depression at time of their initial presentation for treatment." (Bartlett, 1999, p. 270) Depression is a complex phenomenon characterized by low mood, low energy, and low feelings of self-worth. The causes of depression are as complex as the condition and range from psychological events including loss, separation, abandonment, and grief, to use of medications often used in HIV treatment including, but not limited to, zidovudine (AZT), acyclovir, sulfonamides, and anabolic steroids. (Bartlett, 1999; Valente & Saunders, 1997) Stress, life styles, and behavior can also increase depression through the use of alcohol and "recreational" drugs, including street drugs.

Ironically, as the survival rate for persons infected with HIV increases, the quality of life of these individuals is often impaired due to side effects from medications, loss of jobs due to illness and side effects, subsequent loss of financial stability and, finally, loss of belief in self. Additionally, the uncertainty of a life containing psychologically painful exacerbations and remissions of HIV disease discussed earlier, along with the existential realization that AIDS continues to be a chronic, but ultimately fatal disease, may cause greater depression, anxiety, and fear across the continuum of the disease in HIV infected patients. (Brashers, et al., 1999; Selwyn & Arnold, 1999; O'Neill & Alexander, 1997)

The growing chronicity of living with AIDS, along with the fewer deaths due to AIDS, paradoxically, could isolate survivors with AIDS from each other, and from the benefit of mutual grieving processes. (Selwyn & Arnold, 1998) This isolation may be worsened by the fact that those experiencing a longer survival time may increase the time of anticipatory grieving for themselves.

Prognosis

HIV mortality is influenced by new and changing therapies, practitioners' skill and experience in management, and individual patient tolerance for treatment. The fact that HIV occurs predominantly in younger people who can better tolerate the heavy burdens of disease and disease treatments, compounds the difficulty of prognosis. The following factors are correlated with early mortality and therefore may be helpful when evaluating a patient to be appropriate for coverage by the Medicare/Medicaid Hospice Benefit (Stuart, et al., 1996):

- Patient whose CD4 count is below 25 cells/mcL, measured during a period relatively free of acute disease, and who does not have a non-HIV-related co-existing life-threatening disease.
- Patients with persistent HIV viral load of > 100,000 copies/ml; or those with a lower count who have declining functional status, disease complications and have elected to forego antiretroviral and prophylactic medications.
- Patients with life-threatening complications, such as:
  —CNS lymphoma
  —Progressive multifocal leukoencephalopathy
  —Cryptosporidiosis
  —Wasting (loss of 33% lean body mass)
  —MAC bacteremia, untreated
  —Visceral Kaposi's sarcoma unresponsive to therapy
  —Renal failure, refuses or fails dialysis
  —Toxoplasmosis
  —Advanced AIDS dementia complex
- Other factors shown to decrease survival significantly:
  —Chronic persistent diarrhea for one year, regardless of etiology
  —Persistent serum albumin < 2.5 gm/dl.
  —Concomitant substance abuse
  —Age greater than 50
  —Decisions to forego antiretroviral, chemotherapeutic and prophylactic drug therapy related specifically to HIV disease
  —Congestive heart failure, symptomatic at rest

Management of Symptoms

Using a team approach, palliative care will look beyond the scientific quantities, such as the viral load, the CD4 counts, etc., to ameliorate quality of life issues for both patient and family. The palliative care team will address the caliber of life rather than quantity of life for the patient, thus focusing on the patient, not the disease, "Otherwise the age of HAART will end up conspicuously lacking in heart as we run the risk of forgetting what we learned from a disease we could not cure." (Selwyn & Arnold, 1998, p. 902) Palliative care extends from the symptomatic relief of the first psychosomatic assaults of HIV through the protracted trajectory of the illness until the patient and extended family seek end-of-life care for the patient.

The symptoms common to other advanced diseases, such as pain, nausea and vomiting, cough, dyspnea, and depression, are addressed in Table 1 in the section on General Signs and Symptoms. Table 6, which follows, presents interventions pertinent to patients with HIV/AIDS (diarrhea, dehydration, urinary incontinence, skin disorders, and weight loss).

TABLE 6   Symptom Management of AIDS

Symptom	Non-Prescriptive	Prescriptive
Diarrhea	■ BRAT diet (bananas, rice, applesauce, and toast). ■ Determine with patient if symptom develops or worsens in connection with certain medications or certain foods. Caffeine, sorbitol and dairy products are frequent offenders. ■ Maintain frequent skin care procedures to keep skin clean and dry. Use of powders, creams and gels to affected skin areas immediately after cleansing may be soothing and protect from irritation.	■ Diphenoxylate/atropine (Lomotil). ■ Loperimide hydrochloride (Kaopectate II). ■ Camphorated opium tincture (Paregoric).
Dehydration	■ Assess patient's degree of distress and goals. ■ If sweating is part of the water loss, encourage frequent garment changes to prevent chilling. ■ Suggest preferred liquids for rehydration: water, Gatorade, flat rather than sparkling soda, caffeine-free drinks, and diluted fruit juices.	■ Topical lidocaine and/or analgesic/antimicrobial rinses for oral ulcerations. ■ Fluids as appropriate.
Urinary Incontinence	■ Assess for signs of painful spasms or bladder infection. ■ If patient is on oxybutynin, observe for anticholinergic side effects: constipation, dry mouth, tachycardia, etc. ■ Attention to skin care as with diarrhea. ■ Diapers and pads may be considered instead of an indwelling catheter, but the catheter may be placed if there is deterioration of the skin.	■ Oxybutynin (Ditropan) for bladder spasms or neurogenic bladder.
Skin Disorders	■ Be sensitive to patient's embarrassment and anxiety over skin lesions. ■ Advise patient to use sunglasses, sunscreen and protective clothing during sun exposure if on drugs that cause photosensitivity/skin reactions. (Examples: oxybutynin, zalcitabine, saquinavir, plus some tranquilizers and antibiotics.) ■ Application of moisturizers is comforting on skin that is dry or itchy, but without lesions.	■ May need to consult dermatologist. ■ Topical steroids, topical coal-tar preparations, ultraviolet light or sunlight are common treatments.

(continued)

Symptom	Non-Prescriptive	Prescriptive
Weight Loss	■ Assess for signs of oropharyngeal disease that may prohibit swallowing. ■ Encourage high-protein, high-calorie foods; offer small frequent feedings. ■ Have ill-fitting dentures relined. ■ Mouth care.	■ Steroids may stimulate appetite; discontinue if side effects outweigh benefits. ■ Megesterol acetate (Megace) in doses of 800 mg/day may increase appetite, but is costly. ■ Dronabinol (Marinol) may increase weight gain in some patients.
Neuropathic pain	■ Promote skin care (for cleanliness and integrity). ■ Educate patient/family on danger of injury (with potential for serious complications) in patient with combined hypo/hypersensitivity to cold, heat, pain or pressure. ■ Use foot board to protect patient from light pressure of sheets if allodynia present.	Drug of choice is Neurontin (Gabapentin) in doses escalated to at least 3600 mg/day or titrated to effect. Most other agents used for neuropathy lower the serum levels of many antiretrovirals. This may lead to antiretroviral drug resistance.

Compiled from: Kaye, 1997; Smith, 2000; Kemp, 1999; Sheehan & Forman, 1996; Woodruff, 1999; Doyle, et al., 1998; Ferrell & Coyle, 2001.

Diabetes

By Mary Beth Singer

Overview

Diabetes mellitus is the seventh leading cause of death by disease in the United States. (ADA, 2000a) Almost 16 million Americans are affected by this disease though close to half are unaware that they have it. Many times, a person is treated for another disease and is subsequently diagnosed with diabetes mellitus. Diabetes, for many adults, is an undetected illness for many years, due to its nonspecific symptoms. The leading cause of diabetes related death is heart disease, regardless of gender. The incidence of diabetes is rising annually and it is projected that there will be 23 million Americans with diabetes by 2025. (Miller, 1999)

Acute episodes of hyper or hypoglycemia, with complications such as diabetic ketoacidosis and hyperosmolar nonketotic coma require intensive medical and nursing care. As such, for purposes of this monograph, they will not be addressed in detail. Long term complications of diabetes include macrovascular (atherosclerotic), microvascular (retinopathy, nephropathy) disease, and neuropathy. Diabetes is the leading cause of blindness in adults in the United States. With advances made in both insulin therapies and novel approaches to oral agents, improvement in glycemic control has allowed persons with diabetes to live longer, healthier lives. Diabetes is, therefore, a frequent co-morbidity in the presence of other illnesses. Persons with diabetes may die as a direct cause of the disease, or the presence of diabetes may increase the risks for complications leading to death from other diseases. Regardless of the cause of end stage disease, expert attention to symptoms can provide increased comfort and support to patients and families. Many diabetics and their families are quite expert at managing their diabetic care. It is important to their sense of control to actively participate in defining goals for diet, activity and glycemic control. They often can share their unique responses to stress, treatments, or changes over time with their illness. Glycemic control can have an impact on symptoms at the end of life, particularly changes in mental status, visual acuity and certain pain syndromes.

Pathophysiology

Diabetes is a disease that results from the relative lack of insulin or the inability of the body to utilize insulin effectively. Insulin is critical for the normal metabolism of carbohydrates, fats and protein. At a cellular level, insulin binds with target receptors that effectively allows for the transport of glucose across the cell membrane, with the exception of brain cells. (Guyton, 2000) This point is particularly important to the understanding of hypoglycemic (low blood sugar) symptoms. Brain cells use only glucose for energy. Unlike other body cells, which can utilize fatty acids for energy, brain cells are the only cells permeable to glucose without the intermediation of insulin. (Guyton, 2000) As such, it is critical to prevent hypoglycemia. Severe hypoglycemia (20–50 mg/dl.) can cause CNS irritability leading to seizures and coma.

Subtle changes in mentation or frank delirium can be caused by hypoglycemia. In older adults with atherosclerosis, marked hypoglycemia can precipitate acute myocardial infarction or stroke. (ADA, 1999b; DCCT Research Group, 1993) See Figure 19 for a review of symptoms of hypo and hyperglycemia.

In Type I diabetes, the total lack of insulin results in the formation of ketone bodies due to the breakdown of acetoacetic acid. One of the ketone bodies is acetone. Acetone is responsible for the fruity odor to the breath that can occur in persons with diabetic ketoacidosis. Diabetics are taught to test their urine for ketones when blood sugar results are > 240 mg/dl. Infection, missed doses or inaccurate doses of insulin, and stress are examples of conditions that may cause hyperglycemia leading to ketoacidosis. In extreme cases, diabetic ketoacidosis can lead to coma and death.

Diabetes Classification

Type I diabetes mellitus is a commonly occurring chronic illness affecting more than 300,000 children and adults annually in the United States. (ADA, 2000a) Formerly known as insulin dependent or juvenile diabetes, it is considered an autoimmune disorder that results in destruction of insulin producing beta cells in the pancreas. Genetics and viral triggers may also play a role in the development of type I diabetes. Treatment always involves insulin therapy and maximizing glycemic control has been shown to delay or prevent long-term complications such as peripheral neuropathy, nephropathy and retinopathy. Intensive insulin therapy in the form of multiple daily injections or continuous subcutaneous infusion of insulin via insulin pump, compared to conventional therapy, showed significant reductions in retinopathy, nephropathy and neuropathies. (ADA, 2000a) Long term complications stemming from end organ damage, account for the morbidity, mortality and disability associated with this disease.

Type II diabetes mellitus accounts for 90–95% of all cases of diabetes diagnosed each year in the United States. Formerly known as non-insulin dependent or adult onset diabetes, it typically develops over age 40. Obesity is a major risk factor; approximately 80% of people with Type II diabetes are overweight. Diabetes or prolonged hyperglycemia can also occur as a result of other diseases, i.e., islet cell carcinomas and other neuroendocrine cancers, Cushing

FIGURE 19 | Symptoms of Hypoglycemia and Hyperglycemia

Hypoglycemia	Hyperglycemia
■ Diaphoresis, profuse at times. ■ Tremors, shakiness. ■ Anxiety, restlessness. ■ Tachycardia, elevated BP initially, followed by hypotension. ■ Confusion, delirium. ■ Unresponsiveness, coma. ■ Seizures.	■ Frequent urination. ■ Thirst (polydipsia). ■ Hunger (polyphagia). ■ Nausea and/or vomiting. ■ Fatigue. ■ Somnolence. ■ Vaginitis/balanitis (inflammation of glans penis); candidiasis. ■ Type I DM: fruity odor to breath. ■ Unresponsive, coma.

Compiled from Guyton, 2000.

Syndrome, pheochromocytoma, hemochromatosis, or pancreatic disease, or use of medications such as certain chemotherapeutic agents, i.e., L-asparaginase, streptozocin, and steroids.

Effects of Diabetes on Glucose Metabolism

The liver plays a critical role in maintaining normoglycemia (fasting < 110 mg/dl, postprandial 120–140 mg/dl). Insulin allows most of the glucose absorbed after a meal to be stored in the liver as glycogen. Stored glycogen is converted back to glucose in between meals, as needed by the body. This process is called glycogenolysis. Stored glycogen amounts to 5–6% of liver mass, equivalent to about 100 grams. (Guyton, 2000) It is easy to understand how hepatic disease can therefore alter the normal metabolism of glucose. In the absence of insulin, the liver will seek non-carbohydrate sources of glucose metabolism. The presence of insulin in large concentrations inhibits this breakdown of amino acids called gluconeogenesis. (Walter, 1992)

When the amount of glucose exceeds the ability of the liver to provide storage, in the presence of insulin, excess glucose is then converted into fatty acids. Fatty acids are then transported as triglycerides on very low-density lipoproteins (VLDL) for storage as fat in adipose tissue. (Guyton, 2000, Walter, 1992) The resultant dyslipidemia in diabetics has major implications in development of atherosclerosis. (Lewis, 1999)

Effects of Diabetes on Fat Metabolism

The effect of insulin on fat metabolism has major implications for persons with diabetes. Recall that when insulin has induced hepatic cells to synthesize maximum amount of glycogen, excess glucose is synthesized to fatty acid and used to form triglycerides. After being transported to adipose tissue, they then must be broken down into fatty acids and glycerol in order to be absorbed by fat cells. Once inside the fat cells, they are again converted back to triglycerides. In the absence of insulin fat storage is inhibited and fat breakdown or lipolysis occurs.

In response to lack of insulin, immediate fat breakdown occurs, releasing large amounts of fatty acids into the blood stream. Increased fatty acids promote liver conversion of fatty acids into cholesterol and phospholipids. With triglycerides, cholesterol and phospholipids are then transported into blood by lipoproteins. It is this resultant elevation of lipids that leads to development of atherosclerosis in uncontrolled or difficult to control diabetes. (Guyton, 2000)

Effects of Diabetes on Protein Metabolism

Insulin is necessary to allow the transport of amino acids into body cells. It also acts to promote protein synthesis by activating the formation of the many necessary enzymes. Importantly, insulin prevents or inhibits protein catabolism, especially in muscle tissue. Prolonged hyperglycemia or insulin lack causes asthenia through this mechanism of protein wasting. Insulin depresses gluconeogenesis in the liver. Most of the substrates used in gluconeogenesis are amino acids; therefore, in the absence of insulin, the liver kicks on the process of generating more glucose despite serum glucose levels that are high. While circulating glucose is high, lack or resistance to insulin prevents utilization of glucose by body cells and tissues. This destruction of protein depletes muscle and protein stores. Continuous breakdown of protein causes dumping of amino acids into plasma, leading to severe protein wasting which overwhelms the kidneys. Microalbuminuria is the earliest sign of nephropathy in diabetes.

Due to the silent nature of symptoms in Type II diabetes, much of the metabolic derangement mentioned above continues undiagnosed for periods of months to years. This accounts for the high incidence of secondary illnesses such as coronary artery disease, peripheral vascular disease and microvascular disease such as retinopathy and nephropathy.

Other Hormonal Influences of Glucose Metabolism

Several other hormones play a key role in regulating the availability of glucose. Growth hormone, secreted by the anterior pituitary, plays a synergistic role with insulin to promote adequate growth. They are both necessary for protein synthesis and selectively promote uptake of different amino acids. (Guyton, 2000)

Cortisol (adrenal cortex) and epinephrine (adrenal medulla) are increased in the presence of stress. Both cortisol and growth hormone promote fat utilization in the presence of hypoglycemia. Epinephrine has a potent effect on fat utilization, rapidly increasing fatty acid concentration in the blood. They all inhibit the cellular utilization of glucose. (Guyton, 2000) Sympathetic nervous stimulation, such as fear, anxiety, infection, exercise, and shock increases fat breakdown and can increase blood sugars.

Glucagon, a hormone from the pancreatic alpha cells, is secreted in the presence of hypoglycemia. It causes potent glycogenolysis in the liver, elevating serum glucose within minutes. Many insulin dependent diabetics carry glucagon for injection in the event that they have a severe episode of hypoglycemia. Others are often taught how to inject glucagon in case of an emergency. It is supplied in 1 mg and 10 mg vials and requires reconstitution prior to injection. Some diabetics are not glucagon responders.

Advanced Stage Symptoms

Cardiovascular disease, renal failure, and gastrointestinal disease usually complicate the terminal phase of diabetes. Other sections discuss symptoms and care when these diseases are in end-stage. Since neuropathies, retinopathies and infections are quite specific to diabetes, these are discussed below and interventions are summarized in Table 5. Other end-stage symptoms such as nausea, vomiting, delirium, and psychosocial symptoms are covered in the section on General Signs and Symptoms in Table 1.

Nervous System Complications of Diabetes

Long term complications of diabetes significantly impact patients' quality of life throughout the course of the disease. Microvascular and nervous system complications, including nephropathy, retinopathy, and neuropathy, are more likely to develop the longer the individual has the disease and are associated with disease in patients of older ages. Neuropathy of diabetes is peripheral, and affects both the autonomic nervous system (sympathetic and parasympathetic) and sensorimotor nervous system. The loss of nerve fibers and atrophy is progressive and causes significant morbidity and mortality at advanced stages.

SENSORIMOTOR NERVOUS SYSTEM SYMPTOM. The following figure summarizes the deficits and symptoms found in diabetic neuropathy.

FIGURE 20 | Sensory Neuropathy Deficits and Symptoms

Syndrome	Symptoms
Small-fiber damage	Loss of ability to detect temperature Pins-and-needles, tingling, or burning sensations Pain, usually worse at night Numbness or loss of feeling Cold extremities Swelling of feet Pain on light touch (allodynia)
Large-fiber damage	Abnormal or unusual sensations Loss of balance Unable to sense position of toes and feet Unable to feel feet when walking
Motor nerve damage	Loss of muscle tone in hands and feet Open sores or ulcers on feet

(Adapted from Funnell, et al., 1998.)

Assessment should include the use of a pain tool that is specific to neuropathic pain if at all possible. One is described by Galer and Jensen (1997). Another useful tool is the McGill Pain Questionnaire. (Melzack, 1987) Analysis of the patient's descriptors of pain, combined with their self-report of pain intensity using a visual analogue or verbal descriptor scale, guides the selection of a pain regimen appropriate for neuropathic pain.

Neuropathic pain in diabetes includes superficial dysesthetic or deafferentation pain, deep nerve trunk pain, and muscular pain. (Ziegler, 1998) Pain typically presents in a stocking-glove pattern, with initial presentations in the fingers and toes and gradual movement from the periphery to the trunk as the neuropathy progresses. *Allodynia* is an unusual phenomenon seen in neuropathic pain. Allodynia is a combination of pain resulting from stimuli not normally pain provoking (hypersensitivity) and sensory deficit to heat, cold, or sharpness discrimination (hyposensitivity). Figure 20 outlines the various neuropathic pain syndromes.

The chronic nature of pain in diabetic neuropathy has led to health care providers being concerned with addiction in prescribing opioid analgesics for diabetic patients. (Feldman, et al., 1998; Funnell, et al., 1998) There has been ongoing controversy regarding the role of opioid analgesics in the treatment of chronic non-malignant pain. (Galer, 1994; McCaffery & Pasero, 1999) Controversy also exists as to whether neuropathic pain can be adequately controlled by opioids, as long as the dose is high enough to provide symptom relief, or whether neuropathic pain is by its nature resistant to relief by opioids. (Ziegler, 1998) Adjuvant analgesics clearly have an important role to play for diabetic patients with neuropathic pain, but so do opioids in end-stage disease and for patients at any stage experiencing unrelieved chronic pain with other modalities. Hospice and palliative care nurses may, however, experience resistance from prescribing providers who lack a broader perspective of pain management.

FIGURE 21 | Diabetic Neuropathic Pain Syndromes

Pain syndrome	Description	
superficial dysesthetic or deafferentation pain (small fibers affected)—usually intermittent	burning tingling raw searing crawling	drawing electric jabbing ancinating shooting
deep nerve trunk—continuous, may wax and wane	aching bruising tender knifelike	
muscular pain	cramping aching muscle tenderness drawing sensations	

(Ziegler, 1998)

The following figure outlines treatment for neuropathic pain. Please note that several of these medications require starting at a lower dose and gradually increasing to the recommended dose. (Feldman, et al., 1998)

FIGURE 22 | Treatments for Neuropathic Pain

Symptomatic treatment	Drug or Therapy	Dosage
Local/superficial	Capsaicin	Apply topically qid (adequate trial requires minimum of 2–4 weeks)
Systemic: Tricyclic antidepressants (TCA's)	Amitriptyline (Elavil) Desipramine (Norpramin) Imipramine (Tofranil) Nortriptyline (Pamelor)	(10) 25–150 mg qhs (1st choice) (10) 25–150 mg qd (Fewer SE's) (10) 25–150 mg qd (Effects vary) 50–150 mg qhs (Fewer side effects)
Systemic: Anticonvulsants/Anesthetics	Carbamazepine (Tegretol) Mexiletine (Mexitil) Gabapentin (Neurontin) Valproate (Depakote)	200 mg tid or qid or up to 1200 mg/day (blood levels not to exceed 12 mcg/ml. Many side effects and drug interactions. Up to 300 mg PO TID Start at low dose, escalate to at least 1200 mg PO TID 25 mg/kg/day to maximum dose of 40 mg/kg/day at HS or three divided doses (monitor LFTs)
Complementary	TENS, balneotherapy, relaxation, biofeedback, acupuncture, massage, hot/cold packs, PT, psychotherapy	Little data to support specific approaches

(Figure summarizes Feldman, et al., 1998; McCaffery and Pasero, 1999; Ziegler, 1998)

Retinopathy

The initiation and progression of retinopathy in diabetes is associated with the degree of glycemic control over time and also to the duration of diabetes. Other risk factors for retinopathy include age, hypertension, hyperlipidemia, smoking, and genetic predisposition. (Funnell, et al., 1998) Visual impairment to the extent of blindness occurs in up to 12 percent of people with Type I diabetes and 5 percent of those with Type II diabetes. (Hall & Waterman, 1997) The degree of visual acuity for a person with retinopathy may vary daily along with postural changes, lighting levels, and blood glucose. Patients who have had an opportunity to adapt gradually to blindness may function more autonomously than those who have less severe impairments which have sudden onset. (Funnell, 1998) The importance of retinopathy in end of life care is to continually assess for the degree of visual impairment in order to maximize the patient's independent function, and assist with adjustment to loss of vision if it occurs during the terminal phase of illness.

Infections

Infections become more common in the patient compromised by advanced disease and diabetes. Deciding whether to treat infections in the palliative care patient is determined through assessing the stage of disease, patient and family wishes, and the benefits/burdens of treatment vs. non-treatment. Managing infections in the patient with diabetes includes regular assessment and control of blood sugar levels. Stress hormones released during illness or infection can oppose the action of insulin. Decreased oral intake may precipitate hypoglycemia or dehydration. If treatment is not well managed, hypoglycemia, dehydration, ketosis or hyperglycemic hyperosmolar nonketotic syndrome (HHNS) can occur, with a possible need for a higher level of care. (Funnell, et al., 1998)

Symptom Management

Standards of glycemic control as described by the American Diabetes Association (1999) specifically state that the presence of concurrent illness that shortens life expectancy will modify the recommended goal of attaining normoglycemia. For patients with limited life expectancy, rigid restrictions on diet may not be indicated. In some cases, the intake will decrease to the extent that hyperglycemia is not even a concern. Patients, family and professional caregivers should discuss together the goals for comfort and reduction of symptoms. Patients and families may need further education about the stage and prognosis of the illness in order to set realistic goals. Table 7 follows with a summary of neuropathic pain, diabetic blindness, and infections. See Table 1 for other symptom management.

TABLE 7 — Management of Diabetic Complications

Symptom	Non-Prescriptive	Prescriptive
Pain from neuropathy	■ Promote skin care (for cleanliness and integrity). ■ Educate patient/family on danger of injury (with potential for serious complications) in patient with a combined hypo/hypersensitivity to cold, heat, pain or pressure. ■ Use footboard to protect patient from light pressure of sheets if allodynia present.	■ Non-opioid analgesics. ■ Adjuvant analgesics: tricyclic antidepressants, capsaicin applied topically, anticonvulsants, and anesthetic agents. See Figure 22 for specific recommended doses. ■ Analgesics (Methadone or Levorphanol only) when other treatments ineffective (alone or in combination with above). ■ Complementary therapies. See Figure 22 for specific suggestions.
Visual Impairment; Blindness 2° to Diabetic Retinopathy	■ Maintain safety and consistency in environment. ■ Orient patient frequently to where things are located; who is present; and what activities are planned. ■ Maintain independence and functional status as condition allows.	■ Assess for medications that may affect visual acuity (steroids, opioids, anticholinergics). ■ Discontinue medications that may sacrifice any remaining vision. ■ Refer for community resources and adaptive devices if blindness occurs prior to when the patient is actively dying.
Infection	■ Promote skin cleanliness and integrity. ■ Discuss with patient/family how to best meet goals of patient, given prognosis and potential for response. If patient is near to death and has little chance of response to IV therapies, and has chosen "comfort measures only," IV therapies may not accomplish his/her goals. Remember, fever per se is not always uncomfortable. ■ Encourage mobility as long as possible. When no longer possible, turn and position patient to minimize potential for skin breakdown.	■ Treat infection with usual antibiotics, etc. if this will accomplish patient's goals. ■ If treating infection, important to maintain blood sugar levels.

Compiled from: Kaye, 1997; Smith, 2000; Kemp, 1999; Sheehan & Forman, 1996; Woodruff, 1999; Doyle, et al., 1998; Ferrell & Coyle, 2001.

REFERENCES

Abrahm, J.L. (2000). *A Physician's guide to pain and symptom management in cancer patients*. Baltimore: The Johns Hopkins University Press.

Adams, R.D., Victor, M., & Ropper, A.H. (1997). *Principles of neurology, 6th ed.* (pp. 777–840) New York: McGraw-Hill.

Addington-Hall, J.M., MacDonald, L.D., & Anderson, H.R. (1990). Can the Spitzer Quality of Life Index help to reduce prognostic uncertainty in terminal care? *British Journal of Medicine*, 62(4), 695–699.

Agency for Health Care Policy and Research (AHCPR). (1994). *Heart Failure: Evaluation and care of the patient with left-ventricular dysfunction.* Clinical practice guideline no. 11 (AHCPR Publication No. 94-0612). Washington D.C.: Department of Health and Human Services.

Alspach, J.G. & Williams, S.M. (1985). *Core curriculum for critical care nursing, 3rd ed.* (pp. 600–612). Philadelphia: W.B. Saunders Company.

American Diabetes Association. (2000a). Clinical practice recommendations. *Diabetes Care*, 23(S1).

American Diabetes Association. (2000b). Implications of the United Kingdom prospective diabetes study (UKPDS). *Diabetes Care*, 23(S1).

American Liver Foundation. (2000). Web-site: gi.ucsf.edu/ALF/info/topsymptoms.html.

American Thoracic Society (ATS) Standards for the Diagnosis and Care of Patients with Chronic Obstructive Pulmonary Diseases. (1995). *American Journal of Respiratory and Critical Care Medicine*, 152(5), S78–S121.

Bain, V.G. & Minuk, G.Y. (1998). Jaundice, ascites, and hepatic encephalopathy. In D. Doyle, G.W.C. Hanks & N. MacDonald (Eds.). *The Oxford textbook of palliative medicine, 2nd ed.* (pp. 557–572). New York: Oxford University Press.

Barker, E. (1994). *Neuroscience nursing.* St. Louis: Mosby.

Bartlett, J.G. (1999). *Medical management of HIV infection.* Baltimore: Johns Hopkins University, Department of Infectious Diseases.

Bartucci, M. & Bishop, P. (1987). The meaning of organ donation to donor families. *Journal of Neuroscience Nursing*, 6, 369–410.

Bass, M. (1998). Fluid and electrolyte management of ascites in patients with cirrhosis. *Critical Care Clinics of North America*, 10, 459–467.

Batten, H. & Prottas, J. (1987). Kind strangers: The families of organ donors. *Health Affairs*, 6, 35–47.

Billings, A. (1998). What is palliative care? *Journal of Palliative Medicine*, 1, 73–78.

Block, S. (2000) Assessing and Managing Depression in the Terminally Ill Patient. *Annals of Internal Medicine*, 132 (3), 209–218.

Bolla, L.R., Filley, C.M., & Palmer, R.M. (2000). Dementia DDX office diagnosis of the four types of dementia. *Geriatrics*, 55 (1), 34–46.

Borasio, G.D. & Voltz, R. (1997). Palliative care in amyotrophic lateral sclerosis. *Journal of Neurology*, 244 (Suppl 4), 11–17.

Brain Trauma Foundation. (1998). *Guidelines for the management of head injury.* New York: New York.

Brashers, D.L., Neidig, J.L., Reynolds, N.R., & Haas, S. (1999). Uncertainty in illness across the HIV/AIDS trajectory. *Journal of the Association of Nurses in AIDS Care*, 9(1), 66–77.

Breitbart, W. & McDonald, M.V. (1996). Pharmacologic pain management in HIV/AIDS. *Journal of the International Association of Physicians in AIDS Care*, 2(7), 17–26.

Breshanan, L. & Ballou, M. (1999). Palliative care in the home. *HIV Homecare Handbook.* (pp. 337–365). Sudbury, MA: Jones and Bartlett Publishers.

References

Brody, H., Campbell, M.L., Faber-Langerdoen, K., & Ogle, K.S. (1997). Withdrawing intensive life-sustaining treatment—recommendations for compassionate clinical management. *The New England Journal of Medicine, 336*(9), 652–657.

Campbell, M.L. (1998). *Foregoing life-sustaining therapy—How to care for the patient who is near death.* Detroit, MI: AACN Critical Care Publication.

Campbell, M.L. & Carlson, R.W. (1992). Terminal weaning from mechanical ventilation: Ethical & practical considerations for patient management, *American Journal of Critical Care, 1*(3), 52–56.

Carter, G.T., Bednar-Butler, L.M., Abresch, R.T., & Ugalde, V.O. (1999). Expanding the role of hospice care in amyotrophic lateral sclerosis. *American Journal of Hospice & Palliative Care, 16*(6), 707–710.

Celli, B.R. (1998). Clinical aspects of chronic obstructive pulmonary disease. In G.L. Baum, B.R. Celli, J.D. Crapo & J.B. Karlinsky (Eds.), *Textbook of pulmonary diseases, Vol. II.* New York: Lippincott-Raven.

Centers for Disease Control and Prevention. (June, 1999). *HIV/AIDS surveillance report, 11*(1). Atlanta: Centers for Disease Control.

Centers for Disease Control and Prevention. (December, 1996). *HIV/AIDS surveillance report, end year report.* Atlanta: CDC.

Chapple, H.S. (1999). Changing the game in the intensive care unit: Letting nature take its course. *Critical Care Nurse, 19*(3), 25–34.

Christakis, N.A. & Iwashyna, T. (1998). Attitude and self reported practice regarding prognostication in a national sample of internists. *Archives of Internal Medicine, 158*(21), 2389–2395.

Coates, A. (1997). Quality of life and supportive care. *Supportive Care in Cancer, 5*(6), 435–438.

Cooper, G.S., Bellamy, P., Dawson, N.V., Desbiens, N., Fulkerson, W.J. Jr., Goldman, L., Quinn, L.M., Speroff, T., & Landefeld, C.S. (1997). A prognostic model for patients with end-stage liver disease. *Gastroenterology, 113*(4), 1278–88.

Dahlin, C.M. & Goldsmith, T. (2001). Dysphagia, dry mouth, and hiccups. In B.R. Ferrell & N. Coyle (Eds.), *Textbook of Palliative Nursing,* (pp. 122–138). New York, N.Y.: Oxford University Press.

Dardes, N., Campo, S., Chiappini, M.G., et al. (1986). Prognosis of COPD patients after an episode of acute respiratory failure. *European Journal of Respiratory Diseases, 69*(S-146), 377–381.

Desmet, V.J., Gerber, M., Hoofnagle, J.H., Manns, M., & Scheuer, P.J. (1994). Classification of chronic hepatitis: Diagnosis, grading and staging. *Hepatology, 19,* 1513–19.

Diabetes Control and Complications Trial Research Group. (1993). The effect of intensive treatment of diabetes on the development and progression of long term complications in insulin dependent diabetes mellitus. *New England Journal of Medicine,* 982–986.

Doyle, D., Hanks, G.W.C., & MacDonald, N. (Eds.). (1998). *Oxford textbook of palliative medicine,* 2nd ed. New York: Oxford University Press.

Durham, E. & Weiss, L. (1997). How patients die. *American Journal of Nursing, 97*(12), 41–46.

Ebers, G.C. (1983). Genetic Factors in MS. *Neurology Clinics, 1,* 645.

Eckman, M., Harold, C.E., Mauro, E.L., Ninger, L.J., & Priff, N. (1998). Emphysema. In M. Eckman, C.E. Harold, E.L. Mauro, L.J. Ninger & N. Priff (Eds.), *Coping with multisystems complications.* St. Louis: Mosby.

Emanuel, E.J. & Emanuel, L.L. (1998). The promise of a good death. *The Lancet, 351*(2S), 21SII–29SII.

Enck, R.E. (1994). *The medical care of terminally ill patients.* Baltimore: The Johns Hopkins University Press.

Evans, D.A., Funkenstein, H., Albert, M.S., Scherr, P.A., Cook, N.R., Chown, M.J., Hebert L.E., Hennekens, C.H. & Taylor, J.O. (1989). Prevalence of Alzheimer's disease in a community population of older persons higher then previously reported. *Journal of the American Medical Association, 262*(18), 2551–2556.

Faber-Langendoen, K. (1994). The clinical management of dying patients receiving mechanical ventilation; A survey of physician practice. *Chest, 106,* 880–888.

Fahey, J. (1996). *Death out of context; family needs in the critical care setting*. Unpublished manuscript, Salem State College at Salem, MA.

Fainsinger, R.L., MacEacheron, T., Miller, M.J., Bruera, E., & Hanson, J. (1992). The use of hypodermoclysis for rehydration in terminally ill cancer patients. *Journal of Palliative Care, 8*, 70.

Feldman, E.L., Stevens, M.J., & Greene, D.A. (1998). In Veves, Aristidis (ed.), *Clinical management of diabetic neuropathy*. Totowa, NJ: Humana Press.

Ferrell, B.R. & Coyle, N. (Eds.). (2001). *Textbook of Palliative Nursing*. New York, N.Y.: Oxford University Press.

Ferrell, B. (1995). The impact of pain on quality of life: A decade of research. *Nursing Clinics of North America, 30*(4), 609–624.

Finucane, T.E. (1999). How gravely ill becomes dying; A key to end of life care. *Journal of the American Medical Association, 282*(17), 1670–72.

Fox, E., Landrum-McNiff, K., Zhong, Z., Dawson, N., Wu, A., & Lynn, J. (1999). Evaluation of prognostic criteria for determining hospice eligibility in patients with advanced lung, heart or liver disease. *Journal of the American Medical Association, 282*(17), 1638–1645.

Funnell, M.M., Hunt, C., Kulkarni, K., Rubin, R.R., & Yarborough, P.C. (1998). *A Core curriculum for diabetes education (3rd ed.)*. Chicago: American Association of Diabetes Educators.

Galer, B.S. (1994). Painful polyneuropathy: diagnosis, pathophysiology, and management. *Seminars in Neurology, 14*(3), 237–246.

Galer, B.S. & Jensen, M.P. (1997). Development and preliminary validation of a pain measure specific to neuropathic pain: the neuropathic pain scale. *Neurology, 48*, 332–338.

Gallant, J.E. (2000). Testosterone levels. On-line: Johns Hopkins AIDS Line.

Gilligan, T. & Raffin, T. (1996). Withdrawing life support: Extubation and prolonged terminal weans are inappropriate. *Critical Care Medicine, 24*, 352–353.

Goroll, A.H., May, L.A., & Mulley, A.G. (1997). *Primary Care Medicine, 3rd ed*. Philadelphia: J.B. Lippincott. 863–5.

Gresham, G.E., Duncan, P.W., Stason, W.B., et al. (1995). *Clinical practice guidelines: Post-stroke rehabilitation, Vol 16*. US Department of Health and Human Services.

Groër, M.E. & Shekleton, M.E. (1979). *Basic pathophysiology*. St. Louis: C. V. Mosby Company.

Guyton, A.C. & Hall, J.E. (2000). Insulin, glucagon and diabetes mellitus. In *Textbook of Medical Physiology, (10th ed.)*. (pp. 855–856). Philadelphia: W.B. Saunders Company.

Guyton, A.C. & Hall, J.E. (2000). Micturation, diuretics, and kidney diseases. In *Textbook of Medical Physiology, (10th ed.)*, (pp. 405–421). Philadelphia: W.B. Saunders Company.

Hafemeister T.L. & Hannaford, P.L. (1996). *Resolving Disputes Over Life-Sustaining Treatment*. Williamsburg, VA: National Center for State Courts.

Hall, B. & Waterman, H. (1997). The psychosocial aspects of visual impairment in diabetes. *Nursing Standard, 11*(39), 40–46.

Hewitt, D., McDonald, M, & Portnoy, R. (1997). Pain syndromes and etiologies in ambulatory AIDS patients. *Pain, 70*, 117–123.

Ho, K.K., Pinsky, J.L., Kannel, W.B., & Levy, D. (1993). The epidemiology of heart failure: The Framingham study. *Journal of the American College of Cardiology, 22*(suppl. A), 6A–13A.

Hurley, A., Volicer, B., Hanrahan, P., Houde, S., & Volicer, L. (1992). Assessment of discomfort in advanced Alzheimer patients. *Research in Nursing and Health, 15*, 369–377.

Ingham, J.M. (1998). The epidemiology of cancer at the end of life. In A. Bereger, R.K. Portenoy, & D.E. Weisman (Eds.), *Principles and practice of supportive oncology*, (pp. 749–765). Philadelphia: Lippincott-Raven Publishers.

Ingram, R.H. (1994). Chronic bronchitis, emphysema and airway obstruction. In K.J. Isselbacher, E. Braunwald, J.D. Wilson, J.B. Martin, A.S. Fauci, & D.L. Kasper (Eds.), *Harrison's principles of internal medicine, 13th ed.*, (pp. 1197–1203). New York: McGraw-Hill, Inc.

Johnson, R.A. (1999, November 22–23). HIV disease in the era of HAART: Mucocutaneous complications. *AIDS medicine: An intensive course.* Boston: The Partners AIDS Research Center & Departments of Medicine Massachusetts General Hospital, Brigham & Women's Hospital, Harvard Medical School.

Joint Commission for the Accreditation of Healthcare Organizations (1999). *Automated CAMH, August update 1999.*

Kaye, P. (1997). *Notes on symptom control in hospice & palliative care.* (Rev first ed. USA Version). Essex, CT: Hospice Education Institute.

Kemp, C. (1999). *Terminal illness, A guide to nursing care, 2nd Ed.* Philadelphia: Lippincott.

Klein, A. & Kowall, N. (1998). Alzheimer's disease and other progressive dementias. In L. Volicer & A. Hurley (Eds.), *Hospice care for patients with advanced progressive dementia.* (pp. 3–28). New York: Springer Publishing Company.

Knaus, W.A., Harrell, F.E., Lynn, J., Goldman, L., Phillips, R., Connors, A.F., Dawson, N., Fulkerson, W.J., Califf, R.M., Desbiens, N., Layde, P., Oye, R.K., Bellamy, P.E., Hakim, R.B., & Wagner, D.P. (1995). The SUPPORT prognostic model: Objective estimates for survival for seriously ill hospitalized adults. *Annals of Internal Medicine, 123*(3), 191–203.

Kuebler, K.K. (Ed.). (1996). *Hospice and palliative care clinical practice protocol, Dyspnea.* Pittsburgh: Hospice and Palliative Nurses Association.

Kuebler, K.K. (Ed.). (1997). *Hospice and palliative care clinical practice protocol, Terminal Restlessness.* Pittsburgh: Hospice and Palliative Nurses Association.

Lewis, G.F. (1999). Lipid metabolism. *Current Opinion in Lipidology, 10*(5), 475–477.

Long, M.C. (1996). Death and dying and recognizing approaching death. *Clinics in Geriatric Medicine, 12*(2), 359–368.

Luchins, D. & Hanrahan, P. (1993). What is appropriate health care for end-stage dementia? *Journal of the American Geriatrics Society, 41,* 25–30.

Luckmann, J. (1997). *Saunders manual of nursing care.* Philadelphia: W.B. Saunders Company.

Lynn, J., Teno, J.M., & Harrell, F.E. (1995). Accurate prognostication of death: Opportunities and challenges for clinicians. *Western Journal of Medicine, 163,* 250–257.

Martin, F.L. (1992). When the liver breaks down. *RN, 35*(8), 52–7, 61.

Mayer, S.A. & Kossoff, S.B. (1999). Withdrawal of life support in the neurological intensive care unit. *Neurology, 12,* 1602–1609.

McCaffery, M. & Pasero, C. (1999). *Pain: Clinical manual, 2nd ed.* St. Louis: Mosby.

McCracken, A. & Gerdsen, L. (1991). Sharing the legacy: Hospice care principles for terminally ill elders. *Journal of Gerontological Nursing, 17*(12), 4–8.

McDougal, W.S. (1996). The kidney. In J.Y. Gillenwater, J.T. Grayhack, S.S. Howards, & J.W. Duckett (Eds.), *Adult and Pediatric Urology, 3rd ed.* (pp. 617–642). St. Louis: Mosby.

Melzack, R. (1997). The short-form McGill Pain Questionnaire. *Pain, 30,* 191–197.

Miller, V.G. (1999). Health outcomes for persons with diabetes. *Nurse Practitioner Forum, 10*(4), 201–203.

Morita, T., Tsunda, J., Inoue, S., & Chihara, S. (1999). The palliative prognostic index; A scoring system for survival prediction of terminally ill cancer patients. *Supportive Care in Cancer, 7,* 128–133.

Moscardini, C., Tougher-Decker, R., & Ostronski, M.B. (1997). Nutritional needs in the AIDS patient. *Advance for Nurse Practitioners.* 5–6, 34–42.

National Hospice Organization (1998). *Hospice fact sheet* (on-line). Available: *http://www.nho.ogr/basics.htm.*

National Hospice Organization Standards and Accreditation Committee. (1997). *A pathway for patients and families facing terminal illness.* Arlington, VA: NHO.

Newshan, G. & Arnold, D.W. (1999). Palliative care pain and symptom management in persons with HIV/AIDS. *Nursing Clinics of North America, 34*(1), 131–145.

O'Neill, J.F. & Alexander, C.S. (1997). Palliative medicine and HIV/AIDS. *Primary Care 24*(3), 607–615.

Obbens, E.A.M.T. (1998). Neurological problems in palliative medicine. In D. Doyle, G.W.C. Hanks & N. MacDonald, *Oxford textbook of palliative medicine, 2nd ed.* (pp. 727–750). New York: Oxford University Press.

Pirovano, M., Maltoni, M., Nanni, O., Marinari, M., Indelli, M., Zanninetta, G., Petrella, V., Barini, S., Zecca, E., Scarpi, E., Labianca, R., Amadori, D., & Luporinin, G. (1999). A new palliative care prognostic score: A first step for the staging of terminally ill cancer patients. *Journal of Pain and Symptom Management, 17*(4), 231–239.

Pomerantz, S. & Harrison, E. (1990). End-stage symptom management. *AIDS Patient Care, 4*(1), 18–20.

Porth, C.M. (1998). Alteration in respiration; alteration in ventilation and gas exchange. In C.M. Porth, (Ed.), *Pathophysiology concepts of altered health states, 5th ed.* New York: Lippincott.

President's Commission for the Study of Ethical Problems in Medicine and Behavioral Research. (1983). *Deciding to forgo life-sustaining treatment; A report on the ethical, medical and legal issues in treatment decisions.* Washington DC: U.S. Government Printing Office.

Price, R.W. & Brew, B.J. (1997). Central and peripheral nervous system complications. In V.T. DeVita, S. Hellman, & S.A. Rosenberg (Eds.) *AIDS etiology, diagnosis, treatment, and prevention*, (pp. 331–354). Philadelphia: Lippincott-Raven.

Reimer, J., Davies, B., & Martens, N. (1991). Palliative care: The nurse's role in helping families through the transition of "fading away." *Cancer Nursing, 14*(6), 321–327.

Reisberg, B. (1988). Functional assessment staging (FAST). *Psychopharmacology Bulletin, 24*, 653–659.

Reishtein, J. (1993). Liver failure: Case study of a complex problem. *Critical Care Nurse, 13*(5), 36–45.

Rheaume, Y. & Brown, J. (1998). Complexities of the grieving process in spouses of patients with Alzheimer's disease. In L. Volicer & A. Hurley (Eds.), *Hospice care for patients with advanced progressive dementia* (pp. 189–204). New York, NY: Springer Publishing Company.

Rich, M.W. (1997). Epidemiology, pathophysiology, and etiology of heart failure in older adults. *Journal of the American Geriatrics Society, 45*, 968–974.

Rinpoche, S. (1992). *The Tibetan book of living and dying.* New York: HarperCollins Publishers.

Robbins, G. (1999, November 22–23). HIV epidemiology 1999. *AIDS medicine: An intensive course.* Boston: The Partners AIDS Research Center & the Departments of Medicine Massachusetts General Hospital, Brigham & Women's Hospital, & Harvard Medical School.

Saunders, C., Walsh, T.D., & Smith, M. (1981). Hospice care in motor neuron disease. In C. Saunders, D.H. Summers & N. Teller, *Hospice: The living idea*, Philadelphia: W. B. Saunders Company.

Schiff, E.R., Sorrell, M.F., & Maddrey, W.C. (Eds.). (1999). *Schiff's Diseases of the Liver, 8th ed. vol. 1.* Philadelphia: Lippincott-Raven.

Selwyn, P.A. & Arnold, R. (1998). From fate to tragedy: The changing meanings of life, death, and AIDS. *Annals of Internal Medicine, 129*, 899–902.

Shapiro, J.I. & Schrier, R.W. (1992). Etiology, pathogenesis, and management of renal failure. In P.C. Walsh, R.B. Retik, T.A. Stamey, & E.D. Vaughn (Eds.), *Campbell's urology, 6th ed.*, (pp. 2045–2064). Philadelphia: W. B. Saunders Company.

Sheehan, D.C. & Forman, W.B. (1996). *Hospice and palliative care; Concepts and practice.* Boston: Jones and Bartlett Publishers.

Sheldon, J.E. (Ed.) (1999). *Hospice and palliative care clinical practice protocol, Nausea & Vomiting.* Pittsburgh: Hospice and Palliative Nurses Association.

Sherlock, S. & Dooley, J. (1997a). Hepato-cellular failure. In S. Sherlock & J. Dooley, *Diseases of the liver and biliary system, 10th ed.* (pp. 73–85). London, England: Blackwell Science.

Sherlock, S. & Dooley, J. (1997b). Hepatic encephalopathy. In S. Sherlock & J. Dooley, *Diseases of the liver and biliary system, 10th ed.* (pp. 87–100). London, England: Blackwell Science.

Sherlock, S. & Dooley, J. (1997c). Chronic hepatitis. In S. Sherlock & J. Dooley, *Diseases of the liver and biliary system, 10th ed.* (pp. 303–327). London, England: Blackwell Science.

Sherlock, S. & Dooley, J. (1997d). Hepatic cirrhosis. In S. Sherlock & J. Dooley, *Diseases of the liver and biliary system, 10th ed.*, (pp. 371–382). London, England: Blackwell Science.

Small, G.W., Rabin, P.V., Barry, P.P., Buckholtz, N.S., DeKosky, S.T., Ferris, S.H., Finkel, S.I., Gwyther, L.P., Kachaturian, Z.S., Lebowitz, B.D., McRae, T.D., Morris, J.C., Oakley, F., Schneider, L.S., Streim, J.E., Sunderalnd, T., Teri, L.A., & Tune, L.E. (1997). Diagnosis and treatment of Alzheimer disease and related disorders consensus statement of the American Association for Geriatric Psychiatry, the Alzheimer's Association, and the American Geriatrics Society. *Journal of the American Medical Association, 278*(16), 1363–1371.

Smith, J.J. & Kampine, J.P. (1984). *Circulatory physiology; the essentials, 2nd ed.* Baltimore: Williams and Wilkins.

Smith, S.A. (1997). Controversies in hydrating the terminally ill patient. *Journal of Intravenous Nursing,* 20(4), 193–200.

Smith, S.J. (1998). Providing palliative care for the terminal Alzheimer patient. In L. Volicer & A. Hurley (Eds.), *Hospice care for patients with advanced progressive dementia.* (pp. 247–256). New York: Springer Publishing Company.

Smith, S.A. (2000). *Hospice concepts; A guide to palliative care in terminal illness.* Champaign: Research Press.

Stuart, B., Alexander, C., Arenella, C., Connor, S., Herbst, L., Jones, D., Kinzbrunner, B., Rousseau, P., Ryndes, T., Wohlfeiler, M., Cody, C., & Buckley, S. (1996). *Medical guidelines for determining prognosis in selected non-cancer diseases, 2nd ed.* South Deerfield MA: National Hospice and Palliative Care Organization.

SUPPORT principle investigators. (1995). A controlled trial to improve care for seriously ill hospitalized patients: The study to understand prognoses and preferences for outcomes and risks of treatment (SUPPORT). *Journal of the American Medical Association,* 274(20), 1591–1598.

Tamburini, M., Brunelli, C., Rosso, S., & Ventafridda, V. (1996). Prognostic value of quality of life scores in terminal cancer patients. *Journal of Pain and Symptom Management,* 11(1), 32–41.

Task Force on Palliative Care, Last Acts Campaign, Robert Wood Johnson Foundation. (1998). Precepts of palliative care. *Journal of Palliative Medicine,* 1, 109–112.

Taylor, T.N., Davis, P.H., Torner, J.C., Holmes, J., Meyer, J.W., & Jacobson, M.F. (1996). Lifetime cost of stroke in the United States. *Stroke,* 27(9), 1459–1466.

Tong, M.J., El-Farra, N.S., Reikes, A.R., & Co, R.L. (1995). Clinical outcomes after transfusion-associated hepatitis C. *New England Journal of Medicine,* 332, 1463.

Twycross, R. & Lichter, I. (1998). The terminal phase. In D. Doyle, G.W.C. Hanks, & N. MacDonald (Eds.) *Oxford textbook of palliative medicine (2nd ed.).* (pp. 980–992). New York: Oxford University Press.

Ungvarski, P.J. & Schmidt, J. (1995). Nursing management of the adult client. In J.H. Flaskerud & P.J. Ungvarski (Eds.) *HIV/AIDS; A guide to nursing care, 3rd ed.* (pp. 134–184). Philadelphia & New York: W.B. Saunders.

US Department of Health and Human Services, National Heart Lung and Blood Institute. (1994). *Report of the task force on research on heart failure.* Washington D.C.: USDHHS.

Valente, S. & Saunders, J. (1997). Managing depression with people with HIV disease. *Journal of the Association of Nurses in AIDS Care,* 8, Vol. 1, 51–67.

Volicer, L., Brandeis, G.H., & Hurley, A.C. (1998). Infections in advanced dementia. In L. Volicer & A. Hurley (Eds.), *Hospice care for patients with advanced progressive dementia.* (pp. 29–47). New York: Springer Publishing Company.

Volicer, L. & Hurley, A. (Eds.) (1998). *Hospice care for patients with advanced progressive dementia.* New York: Springer Publishing Company.

Volicer, L., Rheaume, Y., Brown, J., Fabiszewski, K., & Brady, R. (1986). Hospice approach to the treatment of patients with advanced dementia of the Alzheimer type. *Journal of the American Medical Association,* 256, 2210–2213.

Von Guten, C.J. & Twaddle, M.L. (1996). Terminal care for noncancer patients. *Clinics in Geriatric Medicine*, 12(2), 349–358.

Wainwright, S.P. (1997). Transcending chronic liver disease: A qualitative study. *Journal of Clinical Nursing*, 6(1), 43–53.

Wallach, J.B. (2000). *Interpretation of diagnostic tests, 7th Ed.* P. 43. Philadelphia: Lippincott, Williams & Wilkins.

Waller, A. & Caroline, N.L. (1996). *Handbook of palliative care in cancer.* Boston: Butterworth-Heinemann.

Walter, J. (1992). *Principles of disease, 3rd ed.* (pp. 272–278). Philadelphia: WB Saunders.

Wheeler, A.P. (1993). Sedation, anesthesia, and paralysis in the intensive care unit. *Chest*, 104, 566–577.

Women's Health Advocate Newsletter. (July 1998). Hepatitis C, the silent epidemic: Who's at risk?

Woodruff, R. (1999). *Palliative medicine, 3rd ed.* New York: Oxford University Press.

Woolfson, R.G. & Mansell, M.A. (1994). Renal failure and dialysis. In R.J. Krane, M.B. Siroky, & J.M. Fitzpatrick (Eds.), *Clinical Urology.* (pp. 314–322). Philadelphia: J.B. Lippincott Company.

Ziegler, D. (1998). Pharmacologic treatment of painful diabetic neuropathy. In A. Veves, (Ed.), *Clinical management of diabetic neuropathy.* Totowa, NJ: Humana Press.

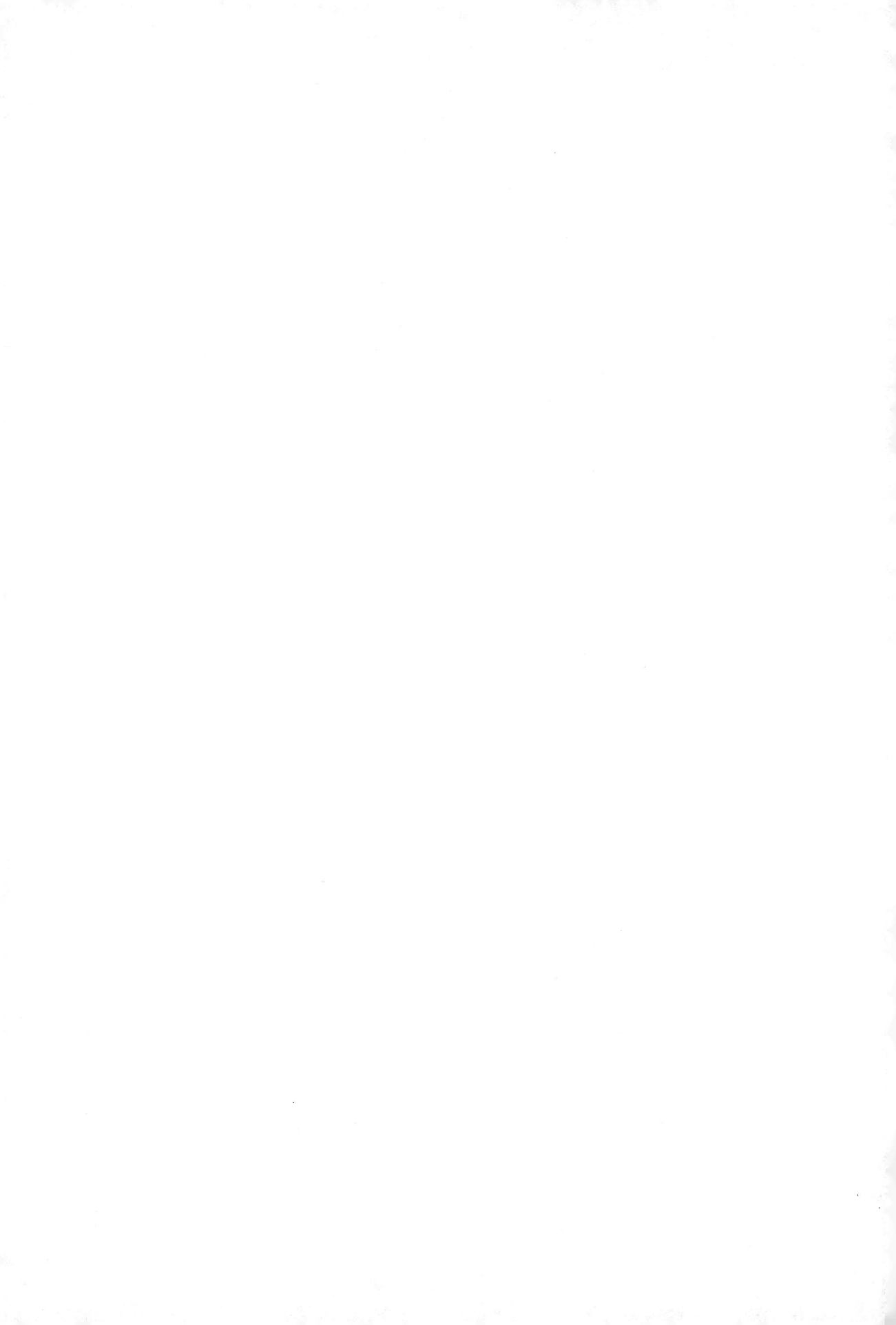